Microbiology
for
Veterinary Technicians

Muhammed Ikram, DVM, MSc, PhD
Animal Health Technology Program
Fairview College
Fairview, Alberta T0H 1L0
Canada

Eloyes Hill, MT (ASCP)
Department of Veterinary Science
North Dakota State University
Fargo, North Dakota 58105

Technical Editor: Joann Colville, DVM
Book Editor: Paul W. Pratt, VMD
Production Manager: Elisabeth S. Stein

M Mosby

An Affiliate of Elsevier

Permissions may be sought directly from Elsevier's Health Sciences Rights Department in Philadelphia, PA, USA: phone: (+1) 215 239 3804, fax: (+1) 215 239 3805, e-mail: healthpermissions@elsevier.com. You may also complete your request on-line via the Elsevier homepage (http://www.elsevier.com), by selecting 'Customer Support' and then 'Obtaining Permissions'.

Library of Congress Card Number: 90-83303

ISBN-13: 978 - 0 - 939674 - 30 - 5
ISBN-10: 0 - 939674 - 30 - 0

Printed in the United States of America
05 06 07 08 / 15 14 13 12 11

Preface

Though numerous other microbiology texts are available, hardly any pertain to microbiology for veterinary technicians. This book was written for veterinary technicians, practicing veterinarians, agriculture students, workers in the biological field and other allied health professionals. It is meant to be used as an inexpensive reference, rather than an exhaustive treatise. Readers may supplement this information with reference texts and journal articles that discuss the subject matter more thoroughly.

I would like to thank Dr. J.R. Saunders, Department of Microbiology, Western College of Veterinary Medicine, Saskatoon, Saskatchewan, for his critical review of the manuscript. Thanks also to Velma Dick of Fairview College for proofreading, and making valuable comments and suggestions. I thank my son Sajid Ikram and Ms. Cynthia Fedoruk for their patience and assistance with typing of this manuscript. I particularly express my appreciation to Fairview College for use of its facilities. I acknowledge my family, especially my wife Zenith Ikram, as well as the Animal Health students, for their moral and intellectual support during the writing of this text. My special thanks go to my copy editor, Dr. Joann Colville of North Dakota State University, who critically evaluated the manuscript for accuracy, consistency and organization.

Muhammed Ikram

Contents

Bacteriology

1

History of Microbiology

How many of us recognize that microorganisms are present all around us? They are present in the air, soil and water, and on the skin, mucous membranes and intestinal tract, and thus greatly affect our lives. Historically, the study of microorganisms has played a major role in the advancement of human and animal welfare. The science that deals with microorganisms (microscopically small living things) is called *microbiology*.

There are several branches of microbiology:

Bacteriology: the study of bacteria.

Virology: the study of noncellular organisms called viruses.

Mycology: the study of fungi (molds and yeasts).

Protozoology: the study of protozoa.

Algology: the study of algae.

Theories of Disease

Before the Christian era, many people believed that an individual's sins were the cause of disease.

Another popular notion before the Christian era was that all diseases emanated from the earth, and were influenced by the stars and seasons.

The theory of spontaneous generation stated that maggots, lice, frogs and even human beings spontaneously arose from various nonliving things. This concept was held until the late 1800s.

The germ theory of disease stated that certain (infectious) diseases are caused by microorganisms. It was proven correct by Pasteur and Koch.

Development of Microbiology

It is difficult to determine specifically when the science of microbiology actually began. It is probably logical to say that it began with development of the microscope.

Anton J. van Leeuwenhoek (1632-1723)

Simple magnifying hand lenses had been used for many years, but high-power microscopy was unknown until Leeuwenhoek used his high-power lenses. Leeuwenhoek demonstrated the existence of incredibly small living objects that could not be seen with the naked eye. He even described their basic shapes.

Francesco Redi (1626-1679)

Redi was the first scientist to help disprove the theory of spontaneous generation. He showed that maggots did not develop in meat if it was covered with fine gauze. He proved this by placing meat in a jar covered with very fine gauze. Flies laid their eggs on the gauze, where the eggs developed into maggots, while the meat putrefied without maggot formation.

Edward Jenner (1750-1800)

He developed the cowpox vaccine that gave cross-immunity to smallpox.

Louis Pasteur (1822-1895)

Trained as a chemist, Pasteur made many contributions to microbiology. Only a few very important ones are mentioned here.

He disproved the theory of spontaneous generation by showing that wine spoilage or souring was caused by bacteria and could be prevented by heating wine for a short time at 55-60 C.

This process is known as pasteurization. He also developed anthrax and rabies vaccines.

Lazzaro Spallanzani (1729-1799)

He proved that as long as food material, after boiling, was sealed from air, no microbes originated in it. This demonstrated that air carried organisms that contaminated food material.

Robert Koch (1843-1910)

He was the first to stain bacteria by adding certain dyes to them. Stained individual cells could be seen more clearly with the microscope. He also perfected the technique of isolating bacteria in pure culture by introducing the use of gelatin and other solidifying materials, such as agar. Development of solid media may be considered one of the greatest contributions of that era.

Koch discovered *Mycobacterium tuberculosis* and reported the isolation of *Bacillus anthracis*.

Koch was also the first to prove that bacteria were a cause of animal diseases. He established certain basic principles known as Koch's Postulates, which were necessary to prove the relationship between a specific organism and disease.

Koch's Postulates state that:

- The specific organism must be observed in every case of disease.
- The specific organism must be isolated and grown in pure culture.
- The pure culture must cause the disease on inoculation into a suitable susceptible animal.
- The specific organism must be recovered from the experimental animal and its identity confirmed.

Though viruses were unknown during Koch's era, Koch's Postulates can also be applied, after slight modification, to viral diseases, and thus remain the fundamental basis of modern microbiology.

2

Microorganisms and Disease

Of all the organisms known, relatively few are capable of causing disease. Infection develops when microorganisms enter the body, multiply and produce a reaction to disrupt normal body function.

Factors Influencing Infection

Infective Dose

This refers to the number of organisms required to cause a disease. It varies with the virulence of the organism involved and the resistance of the host.

Tissue Affinity

Some organisms have an affinity for certain cells and tissues that they may infect and destroy. For example, rabies virus has an affinity for nervous tissue.

Portal of Entry

Regardless of dose, some organisms must enter the body through a certain route, called the portal of entry, to produce disease. For example, *Clostridium tetani* must enter through a puncture wound to cause tetanus.

Toxic Factors

Some organisms produce poisonous substances called toxins.

Exotoxin: Exotoxins are excreted from the bacteria into the surrounding medium. They vary greatly in their toxicity, from very potent to weak. For example, *Clostridium botulinum* produces a toxin that is very potent and can cause severe illness or death after infection, whereas *Staphylococcus aureus* produces a weak toxin causing vomiting and diarrhea of short duration.

Exotoxins are proteins, very heat labile (except *Staphylococcus aureus* toxins), soluble in water, and good antigens. Their toxoids are used as immunizing agents.

Endotoxin: Endotoxins are produced within the cell and are liberated when the cell dies. They are produced by Gram-negative bacteria and are a toxic component of the cell wall. Some of the signs produced by endotoxins are fever, shock, hypoglycemia, diarrhea and inflammatory reactions.

Endotoxins are lipopolysaccharides, heat stable and less toxic than exotoxins.

Enzymatic Factors

Enzymes are organic catalysts and are proteinaceous. The virulence of microorganisms is partly due to their enzymes, some of which are:

Coagulase: This enzyme causes coagulation of fibrinogen in serum, resulting in fibrin formation. The fibrin coats the bacterial cell wall and protects it from phagocytosis. For example, *Staphylococcus aureus* produces it and escapes phagocytosis.

Collagenase: This enzyme is produced by *Clostridium perfringens* and breaks down the collagen found in muscle tissues.

Hyaluronidase: This enzyme is produced by *Clostridium perfringens* and some streptococci and staphylococci. It is also called the spreading factor and breaks down hyaluronic acid in connective tissues, a tissue cement that holds cells together.

Lecithinase: This enzyme is produced by *Clostridium perfringens*. It causes lysis of red blood cells (RBC), and is also found in snake venom.

Host Defense Mechanisms

The animal body has a variety of defense mechanisms that must be overcome by a pathogen to establish infection.

Physical Barriers

Skin: Skin forms the first line of defense and physically blocks entry of microorganisms into the body, unless there is a break in the skin.

Mucous Membranes: The respiratory, digestive and urogenital tracts are lined with mucous membranes that produce secretions that trap most microorganisms and foreign particles, and remove them by their flushing actions.

Chemical Barriers

Animal bodies have a chemical arsenal to fight against infectious agents.

Acidic pH of Stomach: The stomach has a pH of less than 2. Most organisms are killed at this pH.

Fatty Acid Secretions: Populations of microorganisms on the skin are held in check through fatty acid secretion by the sweat glands. Fatty acids have antimicrobial properties.

Lysozymes: Saliva and tears contain lysozymes, which are germicidal agents. Saliva and tears also are a means of flushing out invading microorganisms and foreign particles.

Complement: This is a group of proteins in serum whose function includes enhancement of phagocytosis and virus neutralization.

Interferon: This is a group of glycoproteins with antiviral properties.

Biological Barriers

Attachment Sites: The first step in cell infection by a virus is attachment by the virus, which is possible only if the host cells have surface structures that can serve as attachment sites for the virus. If an animal cell lacks attachment sites, the cell is naturally resistant to the virus. This explains why certain animals are resistant to certain viral diseases.

Normal Flora: Microorganisms normally associated with a particular body tissue are called normal flora. Many of these organisms produce antimicrobial substances and other factors that prevent establishment of infection. When the normal flora is adversely affected, as by antibiotic therapy used to treat disease or by ingestion of a large number of microorganisms such as *Salmonella*, an imbalance may occur and produce disease.

Phagocytosis: This refers to engulfment or uptake of solid particles by living cells. The cells involved in this process are certain leukocytes (white blood cells), namely neutrophils and monocytes (macrophages). They migrate to the area of infection and phagocytize invading bacteria.

Differential leukocyte counts determine the relative numbers of the various leukocytes. These are commonly done to help determine the cause and prognosis of certain diseases.

Inflammatory Response: This is a generalized response that localizes invading microorganisms, arrests the spread of infection, and repairs the affected tissue.

Immunity: Immunity is a naturally protective mechanism. In general, the immune system responds to foreign agents in 2 ways: Natural/ innate or inborn immunity allows each species to resist a particular infection due to the presence of naturally occurring antibodies. It requires no external stimulus and is built into the genes. Acquired immunity refers to resistance to infection developed after birth through exposure to a specific substance called antigen.

Antigen is a foreign substance which, if introduced into an animal's body, stimulates formation of a specific antibody. Antibody is a modified blood globulin formed in response to an antigen stimulus, capable of combining specifically with a corresponding antigen.

There are 4 main types of acquired immunity. With natural active immunity, antibody formation is stimulated as a result of natural infection. In artificial active immunity, antibody formation is stimulated as a result of vaccination with an antigen. With passive natural immunity, antibodies are transferred to the newborn from an immune mother by placental transfer or from the mother's colostrum (first milk). In passive artificial immunity, antibodies are transferred by injection.

References

1. Atlas RM: *Basic and Practical Microbiology*. Macmillan Publishing, New York, 1986.

2. Buchanan RE *et al: Bergey's Manual of Determinative Bacteriology*. 8th ed. Williams & Wilkins, Baltimore, 1974.

3. Cano JR and Colome JS: *Microbiology*. West Publishing, St. Paul, MN, 1986.

4. Carter GR: *Essentials of Veterinary Bacteriology and Mycology*. 3rd ed. Lea & Febiger, Philadelphia, 1986.

5. Pelczar JM *et al: Microbiology*. 4th ed. McGraw-Hill, New York, 1977.

6. Frobisher M *et al: Fundamentals of Microbiology*. 9th ed. Saunders, Philadelphia, 1974.

7. Ross FC: *Introductory Microbiology*. 2nd ed. Merrill Publishing, Columbus, OH, 1986.

8. Whittaker RH: New concepts of kingdom of organisms. *Science* 163:150-160, 1969.

and to each other. For example, bacteria attach to tooth surfaces and reproduce there, producing dental plaque.

The capsule produces infectivity (virulence/pathogenicity). Infectivity is the ability to produce disease. Some bacteria are pathogenic if they can form a capsule and are nonpathogenic if they do not produce a capsule. For example, *Streptococcus pneumoniae* has 2 variants, one that forms a capsule and is virulent and a nonencapsulated variant that is avirulent. Encapsulated *Strep pneumoniae* may be able to resist phagocytosis and thus cause disease.

The capsule prevents nutrient loss and dehydration of the bacterial cell. Finally, it provides antigenicity to the capsular substances and causes production of specific antibodies that are useful in serologic identification of bacteria.

Cell Wall

The cell wall is composed of a base layer and an outside layer. Both of these layers are present in Gram-negative and Gram-positive bacteria. The chemical nature of the base layer is the same in both groups, but that of the outside layer is different.

The base layer is composed of peptidoglycan (murein), a mucopolysaccharide. In Gram-positive microorganisms, the outside layer is composed of teichoic acids that contribute to the

Figure 3. Bacterial structure.

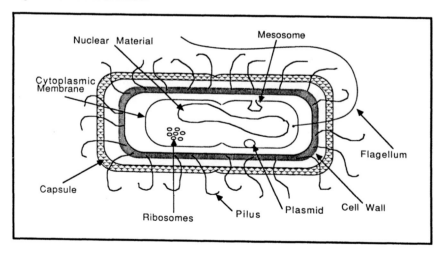

3

Classification and Nomenclature of Bacteria

According to Whittaker's thesis of kingdom classification, the living world is divided into 5 main kingdoms:

Plantae (Plants)

Animalia (Animals)

Monera (Procaryotae): These are procaryotic cells in which the nuclei are not membrane bound. All bacteria are included in this kingdom.

Protista: These are eucaryotic, unicellular microorganisms with membrane-bound nuclei. Included here are protozoa and algae.

Fungi: These are eucaryotic, multicellular, multinucleated microorganisms.

Some main differences between eucaryotes and procaryotes are the following:

	Eucaryotic	Procaryotic
Nuclear membrane	present	absent
Nucleus (within membrane)	present	absent
Mitochondria	present	absent
Chloroplast	present	absent
Golgi apparatus	present	absent

Bergey's Manual of Determinative Bacteriology is extensively used as a reference on classification of bacteria.

According to *Bergey's Manual,* bacteria are classified into 19 parts based on such fundamental characteristics as Gram reaction, cell shape, arrangement and metabolic oxygen requirements.

The scheme of classification used in the eighth edition of *Bergey's Manual* is as follows:

Part: grouping of bacteria based on certain basic characteristics, such as shape, Gram reaction and oxygen requirement.

Order: group of related families having the ending "-ales," *eg,* Actinomycetales. There are only a few orders in the new *Bergey's Manual.*

Family: closely related genera, *eg,* Micrococcaceae.

Genus: closely related species, *eg, Staphylococcus.*

Species: organisms sharing a set of biologic characteristics and reproducing only their exact kind, *eg, Staphylococcus aureus* produces the same reaction to many biochemical tests.

Subspecies: strain within a species. Subdivided on the basis of small but consistent differences, *eg, Campylobacter fetus* ss *jejuni.*

Nomenclature refers to the system of names used in a field of science. The nomenclature for naming bacteria is as follows:

According to the binomial system of nomenclature, each bacterial species name is composed of 2 words in Latin or Greek, *eg, Staphylococcus aureus.* The name need not be descriptive. The first word begins with a capital letter and describes the genus name, *eg, Staphylococcus.* The second word begins with a small letter and describes the species, *eg, Staphylococcus aureus.* Both words are always italicized or underlined, *eg, Staphylococcus aureus.*

4

Morphology and Physiology of Bacteria

Morphology of Bacteria

Bacterial morphology concerns the size, shape, arrangement and structure of the bacterial cell.

Size

Bacteria are much larger than viruses but much smaller than animal and plant cells. The basic unit of their measurement is the micrometer or micron (μ), which is one-millionth of a meter. There is considerable variation in the size of bacteria. The bacteria most frequently studied in the laboratory range from 0.5 to 1 μ in width and 2-5 μ in length. Coccoid forms range from 0.75 to 1.2 μ in diameter. Rod forms have a width of 0.1-2 μ and a length of 2-5 μ. Spirochetes are 3-5 μ long.

Shape

Bacteria can be grouped into 4 groups according to their shape (Fig 1).

Coccus: These are spherical cells. For example, *Staphylococcus aureus*. This organism causes mastitis in animals.

Figure 1. Bacterial cell morphology.

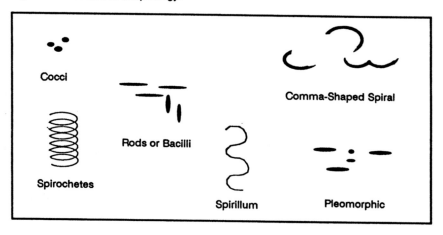

Bacillus: These are shaped like rods or cylinders. For example, *Bacillus anthracis.* This organism causes anthrax in animals and people.

Spiral: These usually occur singly and can be subdivided into loose spirals, such as *Borrelia anserina*, which causes avian borreliosis, tight spirals, such as *Leptospira pomona*, which causes red water disease in cattle, and comma-shaped spirals, such as *Campylobacter fetus,* a cause of abortion in cattle.

Pleomorphic: In this category the morphologies range from cocci to rods.

Cell Arrangement

Bacteria are found in a variety of forms. Some grow as single cells, whereas others remain attached after dividing and form chains or clusters. Many exhibit patterns of arrangement that are important for their identification (Fig 2).

Single: Some bacteria occur singly, such as spirilla and most bacilli (singular: bacillus).

Pair: Some bacteria occur in pairs, such as *Streptococcus pneumoniae* (diplococcus).

Clusters or Bunches: Some bacteria occur in clusters, bunches or groups. For example, *Staphylococcus aureus* forms grape-like clusters.

Figure 2. Bacterial cell arrangement.

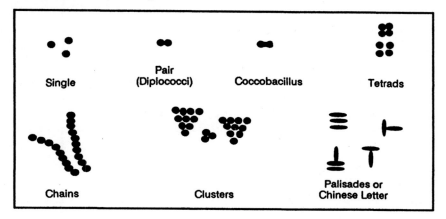

Chains: Some organisms grow in short or long chains, such as *Streptococcus* species.

Palisade: Organisms can be arranged in a palisade or Chinese letter pattern, such as *Corynebacterium* species.

Structure of Bacteria

Careful study with light and electron microscopes has revealed certain definite microbial structures. Some structures are present only in certain species, and some are more characteristic of certain species than others. Such cellular structures as DNA, cytoplasm, the cell wall and cell membrane are common to almost all bacteria. Starting at the outside of the cell and proceeding inward, the following structures are seen (Fig 3):

Capsule

The outermost covering of many bacteria is the capsule, which consists of slimy or jelly-like material. Some examples of capsule-bearing bacteria are *Klebsiella* and some species of *Streptococcus*.

The capsule is largely composed of carbohydrates and/or protein. It has several functions. It protects bacteria against phagocytosis and promotes bacterial attachment to various objects and to each other. For example, bacteria attach to tooth surfaces and reproduce there, producing dental plaque.

The capsule produces infectivity (virulence/pathogenicity). Infectivity is the ability to produce disease. Some bacteria are pathogenic if they can form a capsule and are nonpathogenic if they do not produce a capsule. For example, *Streptococcus pneumoniae* has 2 variants, one that forms a capsule and is virulent and a nonencapsulated variant that is avirulent. Encapsulated *Strep pneumoniae* may be able to resist phagocytosis and thus cause disease.

The capsule prevents nutrient loss and dehydration of the bacterial cell. Finally, it provides antigenicity to the capsular substances and causes production of specific antibodies that are useful in serologic identification of bacteria.

Cell Wall

The cell wall is composed of a base layer and an outside layer. Both of these layers are present in Gram-negative and Gram-positive bacteria. The chemical nature of the base layer is the same in both groups, but that of the outside layer is different.

The base layer is composed of peptidoglycan (murein), a mucopolysaccharide. In Gram-positive microorganisms, the outside layer is composed of teichoic acids that contribute to the

Figure 3. Bacterial structure.

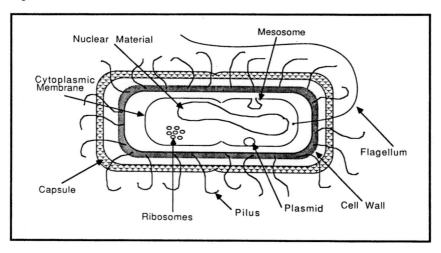

thick wall of Gram-positive bacteria, and of magnesium ribonucleic acid. In Gram-negative microorganisms, the outside layer is composed of lipopolysaccharides and lipoproteins, but no teichoic acid.

The cell wall gives rigidity to the cell and helps maintain cell shape and size. All bacteria except mycoplasmas and spirals have cell walls.

Such drugs as penicillin and cycloserine are antibiotics that interfere with cell wall synthesis and are therefore ineffective in control of infections caused by organisms like mycoplasmas that have no cell wall.

Cell Membrane or Cytoplasmic Membrane

The cytoplasmic membrane is an innermost layer separating the cytoplasm from the cell wall. Its structure is the same as that of the mammalian cell membrane and consists of phospholipoglycopeptides.

It is a semipermeable membrane that selectively controls passage of materials in and out of the cell. It contains several respiratory enzyme systems and performs many of the functions of the mitochondria of higher animals and plants. It has no function in maintaining the shape of the bacteria.

Cytoplasm

Cytoplasm is a complex fluid mass that consists of 2 areas. The cytoplasmic area contains ribosomes, which are RNA-protein particles that synthesize proteins. It also contains granular inclusions, which are primarily storage granules. They are a source of high-energy phosphate bonds.

The nuclear area of the cytoplasm is rich in deoxyribonucleic acid (DNA). The nuclei of bacteria are not surrounded by nuclear membranes and lack discrete chromosomes, mitotic apparatus and nucleoli. Despite the structural differences from the nuclei of mammalian or eucaryotic cells, functions of the nuclear area are similar. It contains genetic information that determines production of protein and other cellular substances. It transmits this information to new cells during cellular reproduction. It has general control of cell functions and is responsible for cellular reproduction.

Mesosomes

Mesosomes constitute a variety of cytoplasmic membrane invaginations. They increase the cell membrane surface area for the purposes of secretion and cell division.

Flagella

Flagella are long whip-like appendages that protrude through the cell wall from a basal body beneath the cell membrane. They are so thin that they cannot be seen with a light microscope without special staining techniques. Flagella are proteinaceous in nature. Not all bacteria have flagella. For example, *E coli* has flagella, whereas cocci only rarely have flagella.

There are 4 types of flagellar arrangements (Fig 4). Monotrichous has a single flagellum at one pole. Lophotrichous has a tuft of flagella at one pole. Amphitrichous has a tuft of flagella at both poles. Peritrichous has flagella distributed all around the cell.

Flagella are organs of locomotion. The number of flagella determines the degree and type of bacterial movement. The

Figure 4. Bacterial flagella.

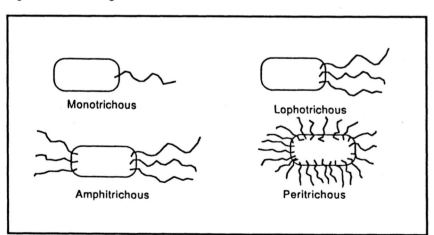

ability of *Proteus* to swarm in a thin film over the surface of some solid culture media is due to the number of flagella present. When flagellated bacteria move in liquid, they generally move in one direction and then tumble to change direction.

Bacteria may move toward or away from light. This is called phototaxis. Bacteria may move in response to chemicals. This is called chemotaxis. When bacteria move into an area with a higher concentration of nutrients, they tumble less frequently than when moving away from nutrients.

Flagella are useful in bacterial identification. They are also antigenically distinct from the rest of the cell and elicit specific antiflagellar antibodies. In the presence of specific antibodies, the flagella are agglutinated and their function is impaired, immobilizing the bacterium.

Pili (Fimbriae)

Pili (singular: pilus) are long whip-like hollow tubes that protrude through the cell wall from a basal body. They are mainly present in Gram-negative bacteria, such as *E coli* and *Pseudomonas* species. There may be more than one present on each cell. They are proteinaceous in nature. Pili can be seen only by electron microscopy. They have no function for motility and can be present in motile or nonmotile organisms.

They act as attachment sites for viruses and mammalian cells. They seem to be involved in conjugating cells and transferring DNA from donor or male bacteria to recipient or female bacteria.

Pili allow bacteria to stick to one another, to other organisms, and to inanimate objects, thus contributing to the adhesiveness of bacteria, a factor that determines pathogenicity. For example, *E coli* must be piliated to cause disease.

Plasmid

The plasmid is a small piece of self-replicating DNA that contains a limited number of genes. It controls conjugation and is called F factor. Many Gram-negative bacteria contain F factor that enables them to form pairs and mate by conjugation. It also contains genes for transferable drug resistance known as R factor.

Endospores

Cultures of a few genera of bacteria form intracellular refractile bodies called endospores or, more commonly, spores. Organisms in the genera *Bacillus* and *Clostridium* are spore formers. Spores have a very low rate of metabolism and can survive for decades without an external source of nutrients. When placed in a suitable nutrient medium, an endospore germinates and a normal vegetative cell capable of growth and cell division emerges. Spores vary in size, shape and location in the cell, and may be classified as follows (Fig 5):

Central: present in the center of the cell, *eg, Bacillus anthracis*.

Subterminal: present near the end of the cell, *eg, Clostridium chauvoei*.

Terminal: present at the end or pole of the cell, *eg, Clostridium tetani*.

Spores are highly refractile, resistant to staining, and heat resistant. They can survive boiling at 100 C for 1 hour. They also are resistant to desiccation and resistant to toxic chemicals, such as pesticides, antibiotics and dyes.

Endospores contain about 15% water, in contrast to vegetative cells, which contain more than 75% water. Starting from the outside, they consist of 2 outer protein coats and an inner DNA core (Fig 6). The outer protein coat 1 has a high cystine content and binds proteins very tightly by extensive cross-link-

Figure 5. Bacterial endospores.

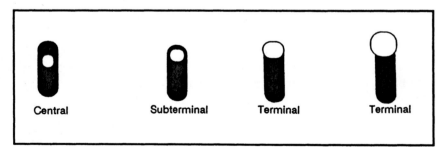

Central   Subterminal   Terminal   Terminal

Figure 6. Structure of a bacterial spore.

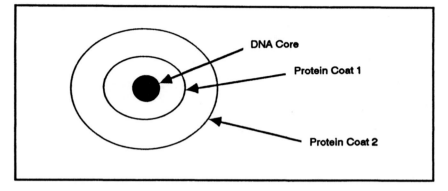

age between adjacent polypeptide chains, making the spore impervious to heat. The underlying protein coat 2 is a cortical layer consisting of calcium, dipicolinic acid and glycopeptide. It is believed that calcium ion cross-linking may stabilize protein against unfolding by denaturation. The innermost core of DNA is well protected by the surrounding layers from heat, chemicals and desiccation.

Sporulation: When environmental conditions become suboptimal, certain nutrients are exhausted, such as carbon or nitrogen, or other environmental changes occur, such as a change in temperature or pH, the bacterium may build a protective core around its nuclear material, forming a spore. This nuclear material, within this protective core, can survive changes in temperature and other harmful conditions that would otherwise kill the normal vegetative forms. Sporulation is not a form of reproduction but allows continuity of life. Eventually the cell degenerates and the spore is released. When a favorable environment is available, the spore germinates and a normal vegetative cell forms from the spore.

Heating spores at 65 C for 15-20 minutes damages the outer coat and permits germination. Placing spores in a rich medium results in uptake of water and loss of calcium, dipicolinate and glycopeptides, stimulating germination. Magnesium is especially effective as a germination agent. Such inorganic ions seem to activate lytic enzymes.

Nutrition and Growth of Bacteria

All forms of life, including bacteria, require nutrients for growth and normal functioning. The essential elements needed are carbohydrates, protein, lipids, water, inorganic salts and trace elements. Other factors that affect growth are temperature, oxygen, CO_2 and pH.

On the basis of metabolism, the bacteria can be divided into 2 groups: Photosynthetic bacteria use light as a source of energy. Chemosynthetic bacteria oxidize chemical compounds to derive energy. There are 2 kinds of chemosynthetic bacteria. Autotrophic bacteria obtain energy from an inorganic source. There are no autotrophic bacteria of direct veterinary importance. Heterotrophic bacteria obtain energy from an organic source. They are of veterinary significance. An example is *E coli*.

Carbohydrates

Carbohydrates serve primarily as a source of carbon and energy. Glucose is the most common source of energy for bacteria.

$$C_6H_{12}O_6 + O_2 \longrightarrow 6CO_2 + 6H_2O + energy$$

Proteins

Proteins serve as a source of nitrogen or amino acids to build bacterial protein.

Water

Water serves both as a solvent and a transport medium for nutrients and metabolic by-products. Most bacteria require about 7-10% moisture in the medium for growth.

Lipids

Only a few bacteria can use lipids.

Inorganic Ions

Phosphorus is necessary for synthesis of phospholipids, nucleic acid and coenzymes. Sulfur is required for sulfur-containing amino acids. Organisms can obtain sulfur from inorganic compound systems. Magnesium is a co-factor for many enzymes.

Trace Elements

Iron (Fe) is required for oxidative enzymes. Calcium (Ca) is necessary for enzyme excretion by certain bacteria and is a major component of endospores. Requirements of other trace elements are less certain.

Vitamins

The requirement for vitamins is not critical to culture of bacteria but they should be supplied if required.

Other Factors Affecting Bacterial Growth

Temperature

Bacterial enzymes are proteinaceous and their action is most rapid at an optimum intermediate temperature. Low temperatures inactivate enzymes and high temperatures denature enzymes. Bacteria have a wide range of temperatures necessary for growth. Temperature-related categories of bacteria are:

Psychrophiles: These are cold-loving bacteria that grow at 0-30 C.

Mesophiles: Most of the pathogenic bacteria belong to this category. These organisms grow at 20-40 C, but optimum temperature for most animal pathogens is 35-37 C.

Thermophiles: These organisms grow best at 40-80 C and may survive pasteurization temperatures.

Gases

Bacteria can be grouped by their gaseous requirements.

Aerobic bacteria grow only in the presence of free oxygen.

Anaerobic bacteria grow only in the absence of oxygen.

Facultative anaerobic bacteria grow in the absence or the presence of free oxygen but must obtain oxygen from oxygen-containing compounds, such as inorganic sulfates.

Microaerophilic bacteria grow best at levels of oxygen less than that contained in air.

Capnophilic bacteria require 3-10% CO_2 in the environment to initiate growth.

pH

The optimum pH for most pathogenic bacteria is between 6.5 and 7.5. Some microorganisms are quite specific in their pH requirements.

Osmotic Pressure

The bacterial cell has a semipermeable cytoplasmic membrane that allows water to pass freely in and out of the cell. Under normal conditions, there is a high concentration of dissolved substances in the cell. The greater osmotic pressure on the inside of the cell keeps the protoplasm of the cell firmly against the cell wall; the cell is said to be turgid. If a bacterial cell is placed in solutions having varying concentrations of dissolved substances, cell turgor changes.

In a solution with a high concentration of dissolved substances (hypertonic solution), water leaves the interior of the cell and the cell begins to shrink. If the difference in the concentration between the interior and the exterior of the cell is not too great, the cell may be able to adjust to the hypertonic solution, regain its turgor, and continue to grow. If not, the cell continues to shrink and finally dies.

If a cell is placed in a solution with a low concentration of dissolved substances or in distilled water (hypotonic solution), water passes into the cell, the cell swells, and it may burst.

A solution containing concentration of dissolved substances in which the cell neither swells nor shrinks is said to be isotonic.

Reproduction of Bacteria

Bacteria reproduce by an asexual process known as binary fission. Nutrients enter the cell from the medium and are synthesized into new cell substances, such as protein, enzymes, DNA and RNA. The cells increase in size, elongate and then become constricted in the middle, after which the constriction deepens, and nuclear and cellular material is redistributed. The membrane with a new cell wall constricts along the short axis and the cell separates into 2 new cells (Fig 7). A newly formed bacterium requires 15-30 minutes to reach adult size and divide.

Bacterial Growth Curve

When bacteria are inoculated into an adequate broth medium at a temperature suitable for their growth, bacterial culture proceeds through at least 4 growth phases (Fig 8).

Figure 7. Bacterial reproduction by binary fission.

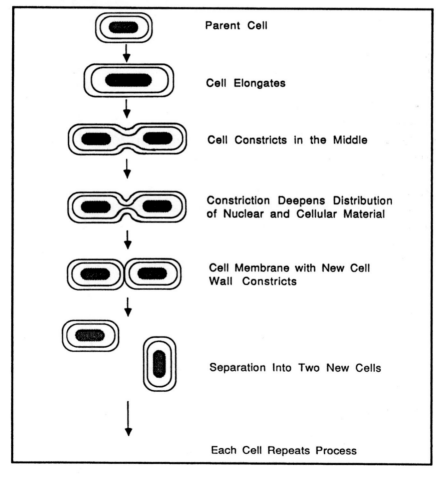

Figure 8. The growth curve of bacteria in culture is characterized by a lag phase (1), phase of exponential growth (2), stationary phase (3), death phase (4) and dormant phase (5).

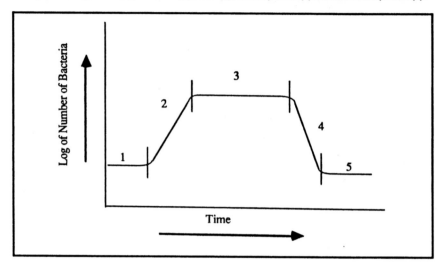

Lag Phase

When a suitable medium is inoculated with a pure culture of bacteria, a certain time elapses before a constant growth rate is established. This stage of adjustment to the medium and temperature is called the lag phase. The lag phase allows the levels of enzymes and/or metabolic intermediates to reach a concentration optimal for growth and cell division. Exponentially growing cells may also show a lag phase if the new medium used for inoculation differs in composition from the previous one.

Logarithmic Phase

During this phase, bacterial population is doubling at regular intervals. When a constant rate of multiplication is reached and cell division exceeds many times the rate of cell death, a culture is said to be in the log (logarithmic) phase. The rate of growth during this phase is maximal and characteristic for any given organism under the particular culture conditions. Cells produced during exponential growth are young, uniform and viable.

Their biochemical and physiologic characteristics are most typical during this phase.

Stationary Phase

Due to the exhaustion of nutrients and/or accumulation of toxic products of metabolism, the growth rate levels off and eventually equals the death rate. This period is called the stationary phase. Bacterial cells are most resistant during this phase.

Death or Decline Phase

In this phase, the number of cells dying far exceeds that of new cells being produced. Conditions that influence the death phase are depletion of nutrients and the presence of toxic products of metabolism.

Dormant Phase

Depending upon the kind of bacterial cells, many cells may adapt to lower metabolic rates, form spores, or go into a dormant phase. Usually few cells survive and resume growth if placed in fresh medium.

5

Laboratory Procedures in Bacteriology

One of the many roles of a veterinary technician is that of microbiology technician. Time spent in this area depends on how much the practice uses microbiologic procedures in diagnosis.

While often it is the veterinarian who collects the specimen, a technician may also do this. It would be likely that the technician receives the specimen and readies it for shipment to a reference lab or prepares it for direct examination by Gram stain or some other technique, and later cultures the sample, identifies any cultured organisms, and perhaps does an antibiotic sensitivity test. The technician may also order or prepare culture media and other supplies needed for bacteriologic work.

Identification of microorganisms is often confusing for the beginning microbiology student. The etiologic (causative) agent is unknown but a tentative diagnosis may help decide what organism or group of organisms to look for. A working knowledge of typical flora and common pathogens of the specimen is helpful.

In addition, subjective judgment is required for interpreting Gram stains, examining colonies on cultures, and interpreting medium changes and other biochemical test results. This is learned through experience; therefore, becoming competent and independent in the microbiology lab usually takes longer than becoming proficient in some other types of laboratory work.

⊃wing discussion will acquaint you with some basic
·gy procedures. The scheme for identifying bacteria to
ed is very basic, but it will tentatively identify many
___   ·rganisms. If you can understand these basic methods
of culture and identification, you can then learn to use more
elaborate systems.

Figure 1 shows the typical sequence of procedures used in
microbiologic examination.

Specimen Collection

Microbiologic examination can provide valuable diagnostic
information if the process is begun with proper collection of
specimens. Improper collection of specimens affects the results

Figure 1. Sequence of procedures used in microbiologic examination.

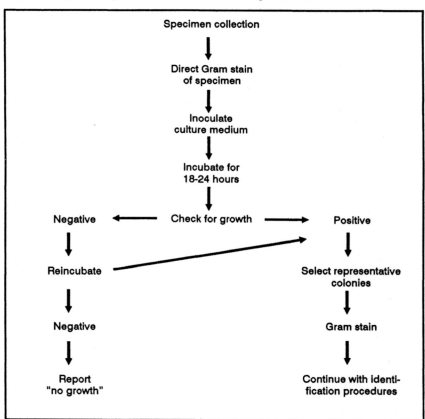

of microbiologic examination and may render culture and identification worthless.

The specimen selected must contain the organism causing the problem. Normal flora and contaminants can complicate sample collection and subsequent interpretation of results. The following guidelines can help you properly collect specimens:

- *Collect the specimen aseptically.* Place the specimen in a sterile, leak-proof container on ice for transport to the reference laboratory, or in the laboratory refrigerator until it is ready to be processed.
- If swabs are to be used for collection, *use an appropriate transport medium* to keep the organism alive until it is inoculated onto culture medium. Special transport medium should be used if anaerobic organisms are suspected.
- Swabs may not provide enough specimen for fungal and mycobacterial culture. *Collect tissue or exudates* if fungal or mycobacterial infection may be involved.
- *Collect fluid specimens in a sterile syringe.* They can be submitted in the syringe if the needle cover is replaced.
- *Collect the specimen at optimal times.* For example, specimens should be obtained in the early acute stage of viral disease and also later in the convalescent stage of the disease. All specimens should be collected before the animal has been treated or after it has been off medication for an appropriate time.
- *Collect specimens from appropriate tissues.* If a certain virus or bacterium is suspected, collect the specimen from the specific tissue the organism is known to infect.
- *Collect specimens from live animals showing typical clinical signs* of the disease being investigated. If the animal has died, collect specimens as soon as possible after death to avoid postmortem contamination by bacteria that invade tissues.
- *Keep multiple specimens separate from each other* to avoid contamination. This is most essential for intestines because of the normal flora found there.

- *Keep specimens cool* until they are in the laboratory, ready for culture. Tissues may be frozen for virus isolation studies but only when absolutely necessary for bacterial culture.
- *Provide complete information with the specimen.* This should include the name and address of the client, species, age, number of sick or dead animals, number of animals in the herd, kennel or flock, type of specimen, clinical history, any treatment given, and results of previous laboratory work.
- *Label the container if a zoonotic condition is suspected,* such as anthrax, rabies, leptospirosis or brucellosis.
- *Obtain the proper forms and specific submission instructions* if submitting the specimen to a reference lab.

Transport Systems

Special transport systems are available for sending specimens to a reference laboratory. Viral transport systems, such as Bartel's (Microscan), contain collection swabs and plastic tubes with cell culture medium, antibiotics, antimycotics and glass beads for cell disruption.

A Culturette swab (Scientific Products) is an aerobic bacterial transport system that consists of a plastic tube with a rayon-tipped swab and a sealed ampule that is squeezed to release modified Stuart's liquid medium. The swab remains moist up to 72 hours.

To provide an anaerobic environment for up to 48 hours, an anaerobic Culturette collection system (Marion Scientific) can be used. It is similar to the aerobic Culturette system but contains 2 ampules. One crushable ampule contains the transport medium and the other an activation solution that combines with a gas-generating tablet to provide anaerobic conditions.

Culture Media

Culture media are used to grow and help identify bacteria. If the specimen is properly streaked onto a medium plate, bacteria grow in isolated colonies that can then be transferred to other identification media.

Characteristic colonies or specific reactions may or may not appear on these media, depending upon the organisms present and the medium used. These observations aid identification of the microorganism.

Several types of media are used for initial growth and isolation of bacteria (Table 1). Blood agar plates (BAP) and MacConkey agar (MAC) are 2 common ones.

Tubes of broth are inoculated for growth of anaerobic bacteria, such as thioglycollate broth, or for growth of bacteria for antibiotic susceptibility testing, such as trypticase soy broth.

Table 1. Some common media used to culture bacteria.

Medium	Purpose	Reactions
Blood Agar	A nonselective isolation medium that supports growth of most bacteria. Used for primary isolation and growth.	Hemolysis by some bacteria: Alpha: greenish zone around colony Beta: clear zone around colony. Gamma: no hemolysis around colony.
MacConkey Agar	A differential selective medium that supports (selects) growth of bacteria in the family Enterobacteriaceae and some other Gram-negative organisms. Most Gram-positive bacteria are inhibited.	Red: lactose-fermenting organisms Colorless: nonlactose-fermenting organisms
Triple Sugar Iron	A medium used to identify bacteria. Colony growth indicates ability of an organism to ferment glucose, sucrose and/or lactose.	Yellow: acidic (fermentation) Red: alkaline (no fermentation) Black: hydrogen sulfide production Bubbles: gas production
Urea	A medium used to determine a bacterium's ability to hydrolyze urea.	Pink: urea hydrolyzed
Sulfide-Indole Motility	Demonstrates hydrogen sulfide and indole production, and bacterial motility.	Hydrogen sulfide production: blackening of the medium Indole production: red ring develops with addition of Kovac's reagent Motility: determined by diffuse growth, producing turbidity throughout medium. If medium is totally black, assume positive motility.
Simmons Citrate	A medium used to differentiate between bacteria that utilize citrate and those that do not.	Deep blue: utilization of citrate

Examples of identification media include triple sugar iron (TSI), urea, sulfide-indole-motility (SIM) and Simmons citrate. Media containing sugars, litmus milk and trahalose are used to identify Gram-negative bacteria.

Two other terms are used when describing media. *Selective media* contain substances that allow growth of one group of organisms and not others. *Differential media* display visible differences caused by growth of specific colonies.

Media Preparation

Blood Agar

Specially prepared blood is added to blood agar base to make this medium. The blood can be from any species, but sheep blood is commonly used because of the hemolytic action by some bacteria, notably *Streptococcus* species, on sheep red blood cells.

The agar should be prepared so that blood comprises 5-10% of the medium. Five hundred milliliters of blood agar make 30 100 x 15-mm plates. Prepared blood can be stored at 50 C for about 2 weeks. Plates of blood agar are kept refrigerated, and remain useful for a few weeks or until they dry out.

The blood is prepared by using an anticoagulant at the time of collection or by defibrinizing the blood after collection. Ten percent sodium citrate at a 1:10 ratio (citrate solution to blood) is the anticoagulant of choice.

Defibrinization requires an extra step, but it is simple and inexpensive. The blood is aseptically drawn into a syringe and aseptically transferred to a presterilized bottle containing a coiled piece of platinum wire and glass beads. Rotation of the bottle for 10 minutes causes accumulation of fibrin on the wire and beads. A 50-ml bottle should have about a half-inch of glass beads on the bottom for defibrinization.

Dehydrated blood agar base can be purchased and prepared according to manufacturer's directions. It is autoclaved for 15 minutes at 15 psi (or a pressure cooker can be used), then cooled to 47-50 C before adding the blood. At this temperature the flasks can be comfortably handled. The blood should be warmed to room temperature before adding to the cooled medium. After mixing the base and blood, the plates are poured immediately.

When any type of plate is freshly poured, bubbles may develop on the agar surface. These can be removed by flaming the agar surface with an inverted Bunsen burner flame.

If only a few plates are used each week, it may be advantageous to use commercially prepared blood agar plates. They may be purchased from medical suppliers or possibly from a local hospital laboratory.

Each batch of plates should be monitored for contamination by incubating an uninoculated plate. The various plates should also be checked by inoculation with appropriate organisms and verification of expected reactions.

MacConkey Agar

MacConkey agar is purchased in a dehydrated form and reconstituted according to the manufacturer's instructions. It is poured into plates and surface bubbles are removed with an inverted Bunsen burner flame.

Triple Sugar Iron Agar

Powdered triple sugar iron (TSI) medium is added to distilled water, mixed and then heated to boiling with frequent agitation to completely dissolve the powder. The warm liquid medium (7 ml) is poured into tubes, and are capped loosely and autoclaved according to medium preparation directions. The caps should be tightened after removal from the autoclave. The tubes are then allowed to cool and solidify in a slanted position to obtain a deep butt and a long slant.

Urea Agar

Urea slants should be purchased commercially because preparing the medium and making the slants are a long procedure.

Sulfide-Indole-Motility Medium

Powdered sulfide-indole-motility medium (SIM) is added to distilled water according to the manufacturer's directions, mixed and heated to boiling for about one minute to dissolve the powder. Five milliliters are transferred into each tube and the loosely capped tubes are autoclaved. Caps should be tightened after autoclaving. The tubes are cooled in an upright position for a deep butt.

Kovac's reagent is used with this medium and may be prepared in the laboratory. Dissolve 2 g of paradimethylaminobenzaldehyde in 30 ml of pure amyl or isoamyl alcohol, then slowly add 10 ml of concentrated HCl. Store the reagent in the refrigerator. Kovac's reagent is also available commercially.

Simmons Citrate Agar

Distilled water and dehydrated Simmons citrate medium are combined according to the package directions and the mixture is heated to boiling. After adding 7 ml of the warm liquid medium into each tube, the tubes are autoclaved. Caps are loosened for autoclaving and tightened afterward. The tubes are cooled in a slanted position.

Inoculation of Media

Aseptic Technique

When inoculating media and handling the specimen, care must be taken to prevent contamination, Sterile (aseptic) technique must be used as follows:

Sear the surface of an organ or tissue with a flamed spatula before it is cut open for sample collection.

Keep culture plates closed except when inoculating or removing colony specimens for testing.

When transferring samples from or into a tube, flame the tube neck before and after transfer of material (Fig 2). Also, do not put the cap down. Instead, hold it between your last 2 fingers (Fig 3).

When flaming an inoculating loop or wire, put the near portion of the wire in the flame first and then work toward the contaminated end. Placing the contaminated end into the flame first could result in splattering of bacteria, causing aerosol contamination.

Figure 2. Flaming the neck of a culture tube before transfer of a sample.

Figure 3. The culture tube cap is held between the last 2 fingers during transfer of a sample.

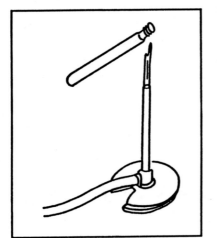

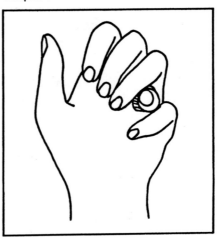

Be sure countertops are cleaned with a disinfectant before and after working with microbiologic specimens.

Plates

Since many specimens contain more than one type of bacterium, culture plates must be streaked so single, isolated colonies will grow.

The swab or specimen material on the wire should be streaked across one edge of the plate (Fig 4). Using a flamed inoculating loop, the specimen is successively streaked from the first area to a second, third and fourth, around the circumference of the plate (Fig 4). Each area is overlapped only once or twice to avoid depositing too many bacteria in an area. Otherwise the resultant colonies are not discrete and isolated.

It is not necessary to flame the loop between areas of streaking; however, be sure to flame the loop when inoculation is complete.

Slants

If agar slants are used, the surface of the slant only may be inoculated, or the butt and the surface may both be inoculated.

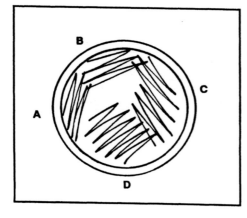

Figure 4. After the swab or loop is streaked onto one side of the plate (A), the sample is progressively spread to several other areas around the plate (B,C,D).

Slant Only: With a straight, flamed wire, touch a colony of bacteria from the primary isolation plate and streak the surface of the slant in an "S" shape (Fig 5).

Butt and Slant: With bacteria on the tip of the inoculating wire, stab the butt of the slant, carefully withdraw it up the same insertion path and then streak the surface of the agar in an "S" shape (Fig 5). There will be enough bacteria on the wire to inoculate the surface even after stabbing the butt. Replace the cap loosely.

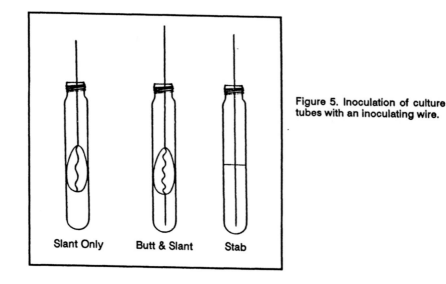

Figure 5. Inoculation of culture tubes with an inoculating wire.

Stabs

Tubes of medium that have solidified in an upright position are stabbed with the inoculating wire (Fig 5). As with the butt of a slant, care is taken to withdraw the wire up the same channel as insertion. Replace the cap loosely.

Broth

A flamed wire is used to transfer the inoculum from the specimen or a plate to a tube of broth. To remove the inoculum, rub the wire on the inside of the tube beneath the surface of the liquid and then swirl it in the broth. Cap loosely.

Incubation of Inoculated Media

Most pathogenic bacteria from animals grow best at the animal's body temperature; therefore, culture plates and tubes are incubated at 35-37 C. Humidity can be increased by placing an open pan of water in the incubator. Culture plates should be inverted so moisture does not collect on the surface of the agar as moisture may cause clumping of colonies.

A candle jar may be used to increase the carbon dioxide content in the culture atmosphere in which many bacteria thrive. The plates are placed in a large jar, a lit candle is put on top of the plates, and the jar is sealed. The candle flame soon dies, leaving a decreased amount of oxygen and an increased carbon dioxide atmosphere. (Note: This does not create an anaerobic condition.) The plates are incubated for 18-24 hours and then checked for growth. If there is no growth, the plates are reincubated in the candle jar for another 18-24 hours and rechecked for growth.

Larger laboratories may have incubators that automatically monitor temperature, CO_2, O_2 and humidity.

Colony Characteristics

An experienced technician can recognize several bacteria based on gross observation of the colonies alone. Various colony characteristics can help identify the bacterium involved. These include size (in millimeters or described as pinpoint, medium, large), color (yellow, white, gray, cream, etc), density (opaque, transparent), elevation (raised, flat, convex, droplike) (Fig 6), form (circular, irregular) (Fig 6), consistency (buttery, brittle, sticky), odor (pungent, sweet, etc), and any hemolysis (alpha, beta, gamma).

Some bacteria cause changes in blood agar. For example, alpha-hemolytic streptococci produce alpha hemolysin that reduces hemoglobin to methemoglobin. The red agar around the colony changes to a greenish color. This type of hemolysis is called alpha hemolysis. Other streptococci produce beta hemolysin that causes a clear zone around a colony, called beta hemolysis.

Some streptococci do not affect the red blood cells of the agar and are called nonhemolytic (or gamma hemolytic).

Stains

Microscopic examination of stained specimens is a routine procedure in the microbiology laboratory. Two stains commonly used are Gram stain and acid-fast stain.

Stained samples may be directly examined for bacteria (presence, numbers, type) and white blood cells. Information obtained from the direct smear may help in deciding the suitability of the specimen for identification, determining the predominat-

Figure 6. Bacterial colonies may be characterized by their form and elevation.

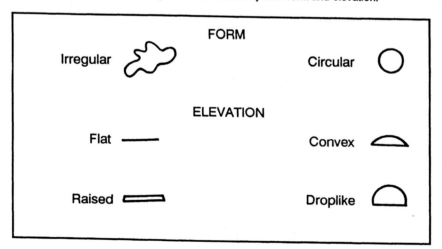

ing organism in a mixed specimen, selecting appropriate media and choosing antibiotics for sensitivity testing.

Colonies of bacteria taken from primary culture plates are also sometimes stained to determine which identification steps are done next.

Gram Stain

Procedure: The Gram stain is the most common stain used in microbiology. The sample should be applied thinly on the slide. Swab specimens can be rolled lightly onto the slide. Touching the sterile wire to one colony on the plate usually transfers enough bacteria to the slide. The colonies should be young (a 24-hour culture), as older colonies may not yield proper results, and often become excessively decolorized.

Bacteria from plates are gently mixed in a drop of water or saline on the slide. If the sample is obtained from inoculated broth, 1-2 loopfuls are spread onto the slide. A smear may also be made directly from the specimen, such as tissue or abscess material.

Regardless of how the specimen is transferred onto the slide (swab, pipette, wire), care must be taken to not destroy the organisms.

The sample droplet on the slide should be encircled with a wax pencil to help find the area after staining. After the material has dried on the slide (it may be held over a flame to speed the process), the slide is passed through a flame, specimen side up, to heat fix the material on the slide. Heat fixing prevents the sample from washing off and helps preserve cell morphology.

The staining procedure is as follows:

1. Place the slide on a staining rack over the sink.

2. Pour crystal violet solution onto the smear. Let stand 1 minute.

3. Rinse gently with water (tap water is acceptable).

4. Pour iodine solution onto the smear. Let stand 1 minute.

5. Rinse gently with water.

6. Wash the smear with decolorizer until no more purple color washes off (usually 10 seconds or less). Do not over-decolorize.

7. Rinse with water and replace on the rack.

8. Pour safranin onto the smear. Let stand 1 minute.

9. Rinse with water.

10. Air dry or blot between sheets of bibulous paper.

11. Examine microscopically with a 100X oil-immersion lens.

Interpreting Gram Stains: The bacteria may retain the crystal violet and iodine and stain purple (Gram positive), or they may lose the purple color and stain red by the safranin stain (Gram negative).

The morphology of the bacteria on the smear is also important to note. The bacteria may be bacilli, cocci or coccobacilli, and may be arranged randomly or in pairs, chains or clusters.

If thick and thin areas occur on the same slide, an organism may stain both Gram positive and negative. If white blood cells, background material or epithelial cells in the thick areas stain purple instead of pink, avoid reading Gram stain results in this area. The thinner areas should give more accurate results.

Determining the Gram stain reaction is an important step in the identification process. It takes practice to perform the procedure properly and interpret the results correctly. To ensure proper staining quality, known Gram-positive and Gram-negative organisms should be stained at least once a week and with each new batch of stain. These control organisms can be kept growing in the laboratory.

Acid-Fast Stain

This stain is used when mycobacteria (*eg, Mycobacterium bovis, M avium, M paratuberculosis*) and *Nocardia* are suspected. Of the various types of acid-fast stains, some are better for mycobacteria and some for *Nocardia*.

Ziehl-Neelsen Acid-Fast Stain: This method uses carbol-fuchsin stain, acid-alcohol and methylene blue counterstain.[1]

Carbol-fuchsin stain is made by adding 0.3 g of basic fuchsin to 10 ml of ethyl alcohol. This solution is mixed with 5 ml of melted phenol crystals and 95 ml of distilled water. Acid-alcohol is made by adding 3 ml of concentrated hydrochloric acid to 97 ml of 95% ethyl alcohol.

The methylene blue counterstain is made by adding 0.3 g of methylene blue (certified) crystals to 100 ml of distilled water.

A thin smear is prepared, the slide is air dried and heat fixed by passing the slide, specimen side up, through a flame. This process fixes the specimen to the slide and helps preserve cell morphology. Ziehl-Neelsen staining is done as follows:

1. Flood the slide with carbol-fuchsin stain and heat over a flame until the stain steams. Remove the slide from heat and let it sit for 5 minutes.

2. Rinse with water (tap water is acceptable).

3. Decolorize with acid-alcohol for 1-2 minutes until the red color is gone.

4. Rinse with water.

5. Counterstain with methylene blue for 30 seconds.

6. Rinse with water and dry over gentle heat.

Acid-fast bacilli (mycobacteria) are stained red, while non-acid-fast microorganisms are blue.

Kinyoun Acid-Fast Stain: This stain is made by mixing 4 g of basic fuchsin, 8 ml of melted phenol crystals, 20 ml of 95% ethyl alcohol and 100 ml of distilled water. The fuchsin is dissolved in the alcohol and the water is slowly added, followed by the melted phenol. The staining technique is as follows:

1. Flood a fixed smear with the stain and let it sit for 3-5 minutes without heating.

2. After staining, follow the Ziehl-Neelsen acid-fast stain procedure.

3. A brilliant green counterstain is sometimes used in place of the methylene blue.

This stain is useful when *Nocardia* species are suspected. they are partially acid-fast and appear as partially stained red microorganisms.

Identification of Bacteria

With experience, you can learn to identify many pathogenic bacteria with the following system (Fig 7).

Figure 7. Flow chart of procedures used to identify bacteria.

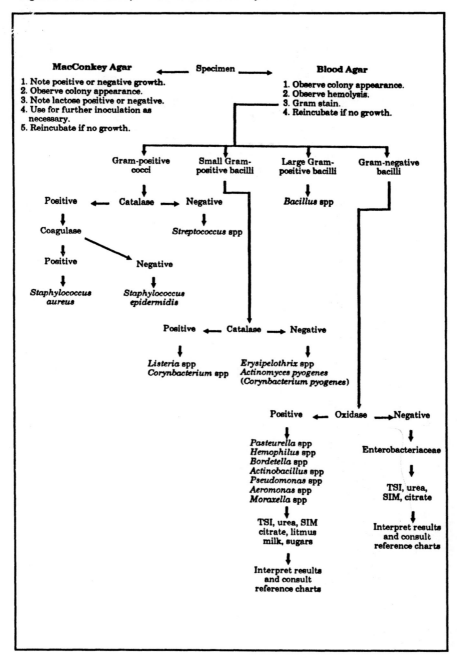

The specimens are first streaked onto a primary medium, such as blood agar and MacConkey agar, and the plates are incubated for 18-24 hours and then examined for growth. If an incubated plate has colonies, you must decide if the bacteria should be identified. There are many points to consider in determining the significance of the growth, and an experienced technician can proceed more knowledgeably at this point than a novice. Referring to lists of normal flora and common pathogens for the different animal species and for the different anatomic sites may be useful.[1,2]

Some of the factors to consider when determining the significance of growth are:

Are bacteria normally found at the specimen collection site? If yes, do the bacteria growing on the plate represent the normal variety of flora or is one type of bacteria predominant? If so, the predominant colony may be the colony to identify.

Is the specimen collection site normally sterile? If so, any bacteria present are probably significant and should be identified. However, they could be contaminants.

What are the colony characteristics? With experience, you can begin to recognize the colonies of certain bacteria, or at least suspect a certain bacterium is involved.

Is there hemolysis? Beta hemolysis usually is significant, and beta-hemolytic colonies should be identified.

What are the common pathogens for this type of specimen? Do the appearance and Gram stain reaction match those of the expected pathogen?

Is the growth due to contamination? This might be suspected by knowing how the sample was collected and handled, and by knowing the colony appearance and Gram stain reaction of common contaminants.

Is a specific pathogen suspected? If a specific diagnosis is suspected and the colony appearance and Gram stain results correlate with those of the suspected pathogen, the colony should be identified.

Sources that may yield almost pure bacterial cultures are blood, cerebrospinal fluid and pus obtained from closed abscesses. Sources that yield bacterial mixtures are sputum, skin, feces and body orifices.

Significant colonies should be Gram stained and the identification process is continued according to the flow chart shown in Figure 7.

Identifying Gram-Positive Bacteria
Media

The specimens are first streaked onto blood agar and Mac-Conkey agar plates, and incubated (see Inoculation of Media). Blood agar and MacConkey agar are called primary agars and are used to isolate single colonies of bacteria for further identification. Most Gram-positive and Gram-negative organisms grow on blood agar. Gram-positive organisms usually do not grow on MacConkey agar, but this agar supports growth of most Gram-negative organisms.

After appropriate incubation, the colony appearance and presence or absence of hemolysis on blood agar are noted to aid identification. Some media, such as mannitol salt agar, are selective for Gram-positive organisms and may be used if a more elaborate identification system is desired. Mannitol salt agar is used for identification of staphylococci. The salt content inhibits growth of other organisms.

A Gram stain on a colony from the blood agar plate shows if the colony is that of a Gram-positive organism, or if the colony is that of a Gram-negative organism that does not grow or grows poorly on MacConkey agar. The morphology of the bacteria indicates which path to follow on the flow chart (Fig 7).

Identifications made after going through the flow chart are presumptive (Fig 7). References should be consulted for further tests to confirm identification. Other factors that must be considered are clinical signs, specimen source and rate of organism growth, all of which can identify an unknown organism.

Catalase Test

The catalase test is done on Gram-positive cocci and small Gram-positive bacilli. It tests for the presence of the catalase enzyme, which acts on hydrogen peroxide to produce water and oxygen. A small amount of growth from a blood agar plate is placed on a microscope slide and a drop of catalase reagent (3% hydrogen peroxide that can be purchased at a drugstore) is added. If the colony is catalase positive, gas bubbles are produced. No bubble production is a negative result.

It is important not to transfer any blood agar with the colony, as blood agar itself can produce a slightly positive reaction. A positive reaction may also occur if a mixed colony was sampled, that is, one with both catalase-positive organisms and catalase-negative organisms growing together. This is why it is important to streak the plate carefully to obtain isolated colonies.

Coagulase Test

The coagulase test is done on catalase-positive, Gram-positive cocci. *Staphylococcus aureus* produces coagulase, an enzyme that coagulates plasma. The test is used to differentiate between coagulase-positive *Staph aureus* and coagulase-negative *Staph*, such as *Staph epidermidis* or *Staph saprophyticus*.

Lyophilized plasma (purchased from a medical supply house) is diluted according to the manufacturer's directions and about 0.5 ml is placed in a test tube and inoculated with a loopful of the organism grown on a noninhibitory medium, such as blood agar. It is incubated at 37 C and read hourly for 4 hours. If the test result remains negative, the sample is incubated again for 24 hours and then read. A negative reaction is no clot formation; a positive reaction is production of clots.

Identification media, such as urea, SIM and TSI, may also be used in identifying Gram-positive organisms.[1,3,4]

Commercial Identification Systems

Commercial kits available for identifying Gram-positive organisms usually are not used in practice veterinary laboratories. They identify organisms to the species or group level, and such definitive identification may not be necessary to establish a diagnosis or treatment regimen for a disease.

For example, the API system identifies 13 species of *Staphylococcus* by using several biochemical tests in a kit. Microscan Staphlatex is a latex agglutination test based on an antibody-antigen reaction. It differentiates *Staph aureus* from *Staph epidermidis*. A BBL Strep Grouping kit identifies *Streptococcus* groups A, B, C, F and G. This system also is based on antibody-antigen reactions.

Identifying Gram-Negative Bacteria

Media

Specimens are inoculated and grown on blood agar and MacConkey agar. Samples are streaked on the plates in an isolation pattern that allows individual growth of colonies (Fig 4). Gram-positive and Gram-negative organisms can grow on blood agar, but usually only Gram-negative colonies grow on MacConkey agar. Not all Gram-negative bacteria grow on Mac-Conkey agar, but most bacteria belonging to the family Enterobacteriaceae grow on this medium. These organisms are responsible for a large proportion of the Gram-negative infections in animals.

Colonies from both plates are compared grossly and microscopically. If it can be determined that only one type of colony is on both plates, then it is acceptable to identify the colony from the MacConkey plate. Not only is MacConkey agar selective for Gram-negative bacteria, it also differentiates between lactose-fermenting and nonlactose-fermenting organisms, another characteristic that helps identify the unknown growth. Lactose fermenters form dark pink colonies, while those that do not use lactose form colorless colonies. This should be noted while grossly examining the plate.

A Gram stain is done on the colonies in question. Gram-negative bacilli are more common than Gram-negative cocci. Gram-negative coccobacilli also may be seen.

Oxidase Test

After the colony has been determined to be a Gram-negative bacillus, an oxidase test is done. Some Gram-negative bacteria produce an enzyme called cytochrome oxidase. This biochemical characteristic is useful in identification.

Carefully choose a colony from the blood agar plate. Do not pick up any of the agar, as blood agar may inhibit the reaction. A colony is touched with a sterile platinum loop (iron-containing wire or nichrome wire may give false-positive results) and the material is rubbed onto a piece of filter paper soaked with the oxidase reagent. With a positive reaction, the paper turns pink and then dark purple or black within 10-60 seconds. No color change indicates a negative result.

Do not use a colony from MacConkey agar, especially if it is lactose positive, as the pink color is confusing with the positive color reaction of an oxidase-positive organism. Strong lactose fermenters are generally oxidase positive.

The oxidase result places the unknown organism into 1 of 2 groups; the identification media used next are the same for both groups in this simple identification scheme. Colonies from the MacConkey plate are inoculated onto TSI, urea, SIM and citrate media.

Urea Tubes

Urea slants are streaked with inoculum and incubated overnight at 37 C. Urea medium is peach colored. If the bacteria hydrolyze the urea in the medium, ammonia production turns the medium pink color. A negative result produces no color change.

SIM Tubes

The tube of SIM (sulfide-indole-motility) medium is inoculated with a straight stab to a depth of about 1 inch. Care is taken to withdraw the wire out the same line as on entry (Fig 5). Hydrogen sulfide production is indicated by blackening of the SIM medium.

Indole production requires addition of 5 drops of Kovac's reagent to the top of the medium. If tryptophane has been broken down to indole by the bacteria in the tube, a red ring immediately forms on top of the medium.

Motility of the bacteria is shown by turbidity throughout the medium. However, if the wire is carelessly withdrawn during inoculation, the resulting growth pattern may be confused with true turbidity, as growth occurs where the wire was inserted and removed. A single line of growth along the insertion path is not "motility." If the entire tube turns black from hydrogen sulfide production, it is assumed the bacteria are motile.

TSI Tubes

Use of TSI (triple sugar iron) medium demonstrates the ability of an organism to ferment glucose, lactose and/or sucrose with or without gas and to produce hydrogen sulfide. The iron in the agar is used to detect hydrogen sulfide production. Formation of iron sulfide blackens the medium.

The butt of the agar slant is stabbed with a straight wire, which is withdrawn and streaked across the surface of the slant (Fig 5). Enough bacteria remain on the wire to inoculate the surface. The cap is left slightly loosened and the tube is incubated at 37 C overnight. The slant and butt reactions are read for an acidic or alkaline reaction, hydrogen sulfide production and gas production. The uninoculated slant remains red.

Slant/butt reactions are recorded as A (acidic, yellow) or K (alkaline, red). An A/A reaction (acidic slant, acidic butt) indicates that glucose, sucrose and/or lactose were fermented. A K/K reaction (alkaline slant, alkaline butt) indicates that no sugars were fermented. A K/A reaction (alkaline slant, acidic butt) indicates that glucose was fermented.

Gas production is indicated by bubbles or cracking of the medium. Hydrogen sulfide production is indicated by blackening of the medium.

Other reactions that may be seen on TSI medium include an alkaline slant (red) and black butt. Assume this to be a K/A reaction. With an acidic slant (yellow) and black butt, assume this to be an A/A reaction.

Simmons Citrate Tubes

Simmons citrate medium differentiates bacteria according to their use of citrate. The slant only is inoculated. If the bacteria use the citrate in the medium, a deep blue color develops. The unchanged medium is green.

After the unknown organism has been incubated and grown on these various media and their reactions read, the organism is identified by its results on the various tests (Tables 2, 3). If the organism's identity can only be narrowed down to a group of bacteria, reference books should be consulted for further identification procedures.[1,3,4] The specimen collection site, patient species, clinical signs, and suspected diagnosis may all be important at this point of presumptive identification.

Further tests for identifying for Gram-negative, oxidase-positive organisms include incubation in litmus milk, trehalose and sugar media. Hemolysis on blood agar and the organisms growth or nongrowth on MacConkey agar are also significant.

Commercial Identification Systems

Use of commercial systems for identifying Gram-negative bacilli is advantageous over use of traditional biochemical tests. The systems are convenient, economical, fast and reliable.

Many of the biochemical reactions used in these systems are the same as those used in the traditional method of identification, such as hydrogen sulfide production, hydrolysis of urea, use of citrate, and indole production. The systems consist of a set of compartments containing different media. They are inoculated and the reactions read usually after 18-24 hours of incubation.

Enterotube II System: The Enterotube II system (including Oxi/ Ferm Tubes) is a commercial identification system commonly used in veterinary medicine. The sample used for inoculating an Enterotube II must be from a pure culture; it is taken from the primary isolation plate, such as MacConkey agar. Two additional criteria must be met: the organism must be a Gram-negative bacillus, and the organism must be oxidase negative.

The Enterotube II system consists of a plastic tube that contains 12 compartments with 12 different media. An inoculating wire runs the length of the center of the tube and extends out the end. To inoculate all the compartments, the tip of the

Table 2. TSI slant and oxidase test reactions.

TSI Reactions	Oxidase	Bacteria
Red slant/red butt (K/K), no H$_2$S production, no gas production	– + + v +	*Acinetobacter* spp (most) *Alcaligenes* *Bordetella* spp *Pseudomonas* spp *Moraxella* spp
Red slant/yellow butt (K/A), no H$_2$S production, no gas production	+ – –	*Pasteurella multocida* (some) *Providencia* spp *Yersinia pseudotuberculosis*
Red slant/yellow butt (K/A), no H$_2$S production, gas production	– – – – – – –	*Hafnia alvei* *Morganella morganii* *Salmonella abortus-equi* *Salmonella choleraesuis* *Salmonella paratyphi* A *Salmonella sendai* *Salmonella typhisuis* (some)
Red slant/yellow butt (K/A), H$_2$S production, no gas production	– – –	*Salmonella gallinarium* *Salmonella pullorum* *Salmonella typhi*
Red slant/yellow butt (K/A), H$_2$S production, gas production	– – – – – –	*Arizona* serovars (most) *Citrobacter* spp *Edwardsiella tarda* *Proteus mirabilis* *Proteus vulgaris* (some) *Salmonella* serovars (most) *Salmonella typhisuis* (some)
Yellow slant/yellow butt (A/A), no H$_2$S production, no gas production	v + + + – –	*Actinobacillus* spp (slow reacting) *Aeromonas hydrophila* *Hemophilus* spp (slow reacting) *Pasteurella* spp (slow reacting) *Serratia* spp *Yersinia enterocolitica*
Yellow slant/yellow butt (A/A), no H$_2$S production, gas production	+ – – – – –	*Aeromonas hydrophila* ss *hydrophila* *Enterobacter aerogenes* *Enterobacter cloacae* *Enterobacter gergoviae* *Escherichia coli* *Klebsiella* spp *Providencia* (some)
Yellow slant/yellow butt (A/A), H$_2$S production, gas production	– – –	*Arizona* (some) *Citrobacter* (some) *Proteus vulgaris*

+ = 90-100% of strains positive
– = 0-10% of strains positive
v = variable reactions

wire is touched to the unknown colony and the wire is withdrawn from the Enterotube. This action simultaneously inoculates all the media.

The wire is partially reinserted into the tube and broken off. The compartments with the wire are anaerobic; the remaining

Table 3. Selected biochemical reactions for some members of Enterobacteriaceae.

	Ind	Cit	H₂S	Urea	PA	Lys	Orn	Mot	Mal	Gluc Acid	Gluc Gas	Lac	Suc
Citrobacter amalonaticus	+	v	−	v	−	−	+	+	v	+	+	v	v
Citrobacter diversus	+	+	−	v	−	−	+	+	+	+	+	v	v
Citrobacter freundii	−	+	v	v	−	−	v	+	v	+	+	v	v
Edwardsiella tarda	+	−	+	−	−	+	+	+	−	+	+	−	−
Enterobacter aerogenes	−	+	−	−	−	+	+	+	+	+	+	+	+
Enterobacter agglomerans	v	v	−	v	v	−	v	v	v	+	v	v	v
Enterobacter cloacae	−	+	−	v	−	−	+	+	v	+	+	+	+
Enterobacter gergoviae	−	+	−	+	−	+	+	+	+	+	+	v	+
Escherichia coli	+	−	−	−	−	v	v	v	−	+	+	+	v
Hafnia alvei	−	−	−	−	−	+	+	+	v	+	+	−	−
Klebsiella oxytoca	+	+	−	+	−	+	−	−	+	+	+	+	+
Klebsiella pneumoniae ss pneumoniae	−	+	−	+	−	+	−	−	+	+	+	+	+
Morganella morganii	+	−	−	+	+	−	+	+	−	+	v	−	−
Proteus mirabilis	−	v	+	+	+	−	+	+	−	+	+	−	v
Proteus vulgaris	+	v	+	+	+	−	−	+	−	+	+	−	+
Providencia alcalifaciens	+	+	−	−	+	−	−	+	−	+	v	−	v
Providencia stuartii	+	+	−	v	+	−	−	v	−	+	+	−	v
Salmonella spp	−	+	+	−	−	+	+	+	−	+	+	−	−
Serratia liquefaciens	−	+	−	−	−	+	+	+	−	+	v	−	+
Serratia marcescens	−	+	−	v	−	+	+	+	−	+	v	−	+
Serratia rubidaea	−	+	−	−	−	v	−	v	v	+	v	+	+
Yersinia enterocolitica	v	−	−	v	−	−	+	−	−	+	−	−	+
Yersinia pseudotuberculosis	−	−	−	+	−	−	−	−	−	+	−	−	−

+ = 90-100% of strains positive
− = 0-10% of strains positive
v = variable reaction

Ind = indole
Cit = citrate
H₂S = hydrogen sulfide
Urea = urease

PA = phenylalanine deaminase
Lys = lysine
Orn = ornithine
Mot = motility
Mal = malonate
Gluc = glucose
Lac = lactose
Suc = sucrose

compartments are aerobic once a plastic strip on the side of the tube has been removed.

After incubation at 35-37 C for 18-24 hours, the media reactions are read and recorded on a special form. Positive reactions have certain values, and the sum of these results is recorded as a 5-digit code. This code number is then located in a manual that lists the scientific name of the unknown organism.

If the Gram-negative bacillus is oxidase positive, the Oxi/ Ferm Tube can be used. It consists of 9 standard biochemical tests. The results are read and used according to the computer code and identification system.

Other Commercial Kits: Another commonly used system is the API20E system, which identifies both oxidase-negative and oxidase-positive Gram-negative bacilli. Its use makes identification of unknowns simple and concise. Many other commercial kits are available and are listed in the catalogs of such distributors as Scientific Products.

Automated Systems

Automated systems can provide Gram-positive and Gram-negative identification, anaerobe and yeast identification, and susceptibility test results in less time than with traditional methods. For example, after the organism has been cultured and isolated, many identifications and susceptibilities can be obtained within 4-6 hours. The principles for identification are similar to those for traditional methods using biochemical tests, but the instrument measures the chemical interactions between substrate and sample instead of the technician's reading them visually. The Vitek System (McDonnell Douglas Health Systems) is one such instrument. Another instrument, the Microbial Identification System, identifies organisms by determining their fatty acid composition.

Antimicrobial Susceptibility Testing

When bacteria are isolated from a patient, an antimicrobial susceptibility test is done to determine the susceptibility or resistance of the bacteria to antimicrobial drugs. The results of this test can indicate which antimicrobial to use in treatment.

The specimen used for antimicrobial susceptibility testing should be taken from the animal before any antimicrobial treatment begins. The veterinarian may begin drug therapy before obtaining the susceptibility results, but may change to a more appropriate drug when the results are available.

Rather than use fresh clinical material for a direct susceptibility test, it is better to first isolate the suspected pathogen and then do the susceptibility testing. This ensures that the test is not done on a mixed floral specimen or on a contaminant, but rather on the causative organism. A Gram stain is done on the isolate to determine which antimicrobial discs to use. Some antimicrobials are more effective against Gram-positive or Gram-negative bacteria. Groups of antimicrobials may also be tested according to the disease being investigated, such as respiratory disease or mastitis. Each typically responds to certain groups of antimicrobials.

Disc Diffusion Method

The Bauer-Kirby technique for antimicrobial susceptibility testing is widely accepted in veterinary medicine. After 1-3 colonies of the isolated bacteria are added to 4 ml of trypticase soy broth, the broth is incubated at 37 C for several hours until moderate turbidity develops. The degree of turbidity is compared to that of a barium sulfate standard. (The standard consists of 0.5 ml of 1% barium chloride and 99.5 ml of 1% sulfuric acid.) The broth is reincubated or diluted with sterile saline until the turbidities of the broth and the standard are the same. The bacterial suspension is then ready to plate onto Mueller-Hinton agar. It is important to use a bacterial suspension of the correct turbidity, as the sizes of zones of inhibited growth (see below) have been determined using suspensions with turbidity equal to that of the standard.

Mueller-Hinton agar must be used for the susceptibility test. Standard sizes of zones of inhibited growth have been established using this medium and are not applicable to other kinds of media, such as blood agar. A sterile cotton swab is placed into the trypticase soy broth, excess broth is squeezed out by pressing the swab against the side of the tube and the swab is then streaked onto the entire surface of the Mueller-Hinton plate in 2-3 directions (Fig 8).

Several antimicrobial discs can be placed on the agar, but their centers must be at least 24 mm apart and the discs 10 mm from the edge of the plate. Each disc is gently pressed onto the agar surface, the plate cover is replaced, and the plate inverted and incubated for 16-24 hours at 37 C.

The antimicrobial drug in each disc diffuses out into the agar. If the bacteria growing on the surface of the agar are susceptible to the antimicrobial agent, there will be no bacterial growth around the disc. This area of no bacterial growth is called a zone of inhibition. Diffusion of the drug into the agar inhibits growth of bacteria.

On the other hand, if the bacteria are resistant to the drug, the bacteria grow up to the edge of the disc. This indicates that the drug cannot inhibit growth of the bacteria.

There can be varying degrees of susceptibility; therefore, the zone of inhibition around the disc is measured and compared to established zone sizes for that drug. The diameters of the zones are read to the nearest millimeter. In this way, bacteria are classified as resistant, intermediate or susceptible (R,I,S) to the various drugs tested.

One other effect that may be seen is a distinct zone around a disc, but consisting of light bacterial growth. There are 2 possible causes for this effect. Some sulfa drugs display this phenomenon. Also, *Proteus* species may develop swarming growth that lightly covers the zone. In both cases, the zone diameter is measured and the growth is ignored.

Broth Dilution Tests

Susceptibility testing as described above shows inhibition of bacterial growth by antimicrobials but it cannot differentiate between bacteriostatic (inhibiting bacterial proliferation) or bactericidal (killing of bacteria) effects. To do this, broth dilution tests can be done to determine the minimal inhibitory

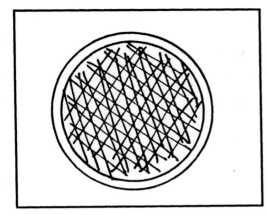

Figure 8. In antimicrobial susceptibility testing, the sample is incubated in trypticase soy broth, and
then a swab sample is streaked in
several directions onto Mueller-
Hinton agar.

concentration (MIC) and the minimal bactericidal concentration
(MBC) of antimicrobial drugs.

MIC: The MIC test consists of a series of test wells containing
decreasing concentrations of a particular antimicrobial drug.
Each well is inoculated with the test organism. The lowest
concentration that prevents visible growth is the MIC.

MBC: To determine if the drug is bactericidal, the material
from the wells that show no visible growth is inoculated into
drug-free broth. If growth then occurs in this broth, the drug
was only bacteriostatic. If no growth occurs, the antimicrobial
has killed the bacteria and is bactericidal. The MBC has been
determined.

Identifying Anaerobic Bacteria

Anaerobes are microorganisms that live and grow in the
absence of oxygen in their environment. They are normal flora
in the oral cavity and gastrointestinal, genitourinary and upper
respiratory tracts. Some of these bacteria are also potential
pathogens. They can cause infections in any area of the body,
such as abscesses, wound infections, gangrenous conditions,
dental infections and reproductive tract infections.

To successfully isolate and identify strict anaerobes (bacteria
that only grow in the absence of oxygen), the specimen should
be protected from oxygen during collection, inoculation and
incubation. In addition, an increased carbon dioxide atmosphere

is optimal for some anaerobic growth, and special media may also be required.

When transporting the specimen to the laboratory, aspirated samples are sometimes submitted in the syringe with the needle inserted into a rubber stopper to maintain an anaerobic environment. Special anaerobic transport bottles, vials or tubes also can be used.

Collection of the specimen by swab increases the chance of exposure to oxygen. Transport tubes containing reduced medium tend to protect oxygen-sensitive microbes on swab samples.

A piece of infected tissue is a good specimen to submit for anaerobic culture. Anaerobes survive longer in tissue specimens than on swabs.

Gram-stained smears of infected specimens may show Gram-positive or Gram-negative organisms. Anaerobes are found in both groups.

The specimen is inoculated onto a blood agar plate and into thioglycollate broth, a liquid medium used to grow anaerobes. The blood agar plates are put into an anaerobe jar, which provides an anaerobic environment during incubation. A self-contained system, such as Gas Pak (Becton Dickinson), can be used. It consists of a sealable jar and chemicals to produce an anaerobic atmosphere with increased carbon dioxide. An indicator strip placed inside the jar turns colorless in the absence of oxygen. Disposable systems are also available.

The inoculated plates are placed inside the jar, water is added to the chemical envelope to start the reactions, and the jar is sealed and put in a 37-C incubator for 48 hours before checking for growth. Anaerobes usually grow more slowly than aerobes.

Twenty-four hours after inoculation, a sample from the thioglycollate broth is streaked onto a blood agar plate. Fastidious organisms may have grown in this broth that would not grow when the specimen was inoculated directly on a blood agar plate.

Reference books should be consulted for identification of anaerobes.[1,3,4] The procedures are similar to those used for aerobic bacteria, but the media and tests may not be the same.

Procedures to identify anaerobes must be done anaerobically, just as with their isolation. A commercial system, such as the API Anaerobic Strip, is available.

Testing Milk for Mastitis

A veterinary technician should be familiar with tests performed on milk, especially if the clinic does any dairy work. Dairymen may belong to the Dairy Herd Improvement Association (DHIA) and sell their milk to a creamery, both of which test the milk. Mastitis testing is emphasized in the following discussion, but other tests are also mentioned.

Quality-Control Tests

Quality-control tests on milk samples include tests for the presence of antibiotics, phosphatase, sediment, added water, coliforms and other bacteria, solids not fat, protein, butterfat and somatic cells. Culturing milk for bacteria can be accomplished by routine methods.

The presence of somatic cells is the basis for mastitis tests. Somatic cells are body cells usually associated with inflammation in the udder. Neutrophils are primary cells seen, but other white blood cells and body cells are also counted in the confirmatory tests if they are present. Counts of greater than 500,000 cells/ml of milk indicate mastitis or other abnormalities. These tests are not used for diagnosis of mastitis, as other conditions can also cause an increase in the somatic cell concentration.

Screening Tests

Screening tests frequently used are the California mastitis test, the Wisconsin mastitis test and the Whirl-Flo strip cup.

California Mastitis Test: This test is a qualitative screening test for mastitis that can be used as a cowside test. If the test cannot be done immediately, the milk can be refrigerated for up to 36 hours. Before testing, the milk must be well mixed, as the cells that react with the reagent tend to migrate with milkfat.

The test reagent is a detergent that reacts with the DNA of the nuclei of the leukocytes present in the mastitic milk. Milk from each quarter is drawn into 4 wells on a testing paddle. The test reagent solution is added to the cups in roughly a 1:1 ratio and the paddle is swirled. A strongly positive mastitis sample forms a thick gel, while a negative sample remains liquid. Varying degrees of precipitation also occur, and the reaction is graded accordingly.

Wisconsin Mastitis Test: The Wisconsin mastitis test quantitatively measures the viscosity of a milk-detergent mixture. As in the California mastitis test, the mixture becomes viscous to varying degrees if there are leukocytes in the milk. This test allows a more objective way of grading the reaction than with the California mastitis test.

The requirements of this test are specific. Refrigerated milk samples must be tested within 36 hours after collection. Measured amounts of milk and reagent are dispensed into special test tubes and mixed by a uniform technique. A special measuring square is then used to measure the fluid portion remaining in each tube, which is an indication of viscosity.

Whirl-Flo Strip Cup: This is another cowside screening test that can detect early mastitis. It consists of running a stream of milk down a tilted black plastic strip. Abnormal milk shows specks of white flakes, small milk curds and a watery consistency. These are all gross signs of mastitis.

Confirmatory Tests: Confirmatory tests frequently performed are the direct microscopic somatic cell count, electronic somatic cell count and the automated fluorescent dye somatic cell count.

Direct Microscopic Somatic Cell Count: This is a manual method of counting the somatic cells in a milk sample. A certain volume of milk is smeared onto a slide and stained with a milk smear stain. The cells are counted microscopically and reported as the number of somatic cells per milliliter.

Electronic Somatic Cell Count: Electronic cell counters (Coulter Electronics) have been used to count the somatic cells in milk samples. A cell-fixing solution is first added to the milk, followed by a diluent that also dissolves the fat. The sample is heated and run through the instrument. Results are reported as the cell count per milliliter of milk.

Fluorescent Dye Somatic Cell Count: The Fossamatic 215 (Dickey-John) is an instrument used for somatic cell counts in milk. With this automated method, a fluorescent dye is added to a milk sample. The dye forms a complex with the nuclei of the somatic cells and fluoresces under ultraviolet light. The sample is sprayed onto a rotating disc and illuminated by an ultraviolet lamp, causing the cells to fluoresce. Each fluorescing cell produces an electrical pulse that is counted by the instrument as one cell.

References

1. Carter GR: *Diagnostic Procedures in Veterinary Bacteriology and Mycology*. 4th ed. Charles C Thomas, Springfield, IL, 1984.

2. McCurnin DM: *Clinical Textbook for Veterinary Technicians*. Saunders, Philadelphia, 1985.

3. Carter ME, in Pratt PW: *Laboratory Procedures for Animal Health Technicians*. American Veterinary Publications, Goleta, CA, 1985.

4. Finegold SM and Martin WJ: *Diagnostic Microbiology*. 6th ed. Mosby, St. Louis, 1982.

6

Gram-Positive Cocci

Family: Micrococcaceae
Genus: *Staphylococcus*

This is the only pathogenic member of this family.

General Characteristics

Staphylococcus organisms are Gram-positive cocci occurring in grape-like clusters or bunches. They are nonmotile, catalase positive, nonspore forming, aerobic or facultatively anaerobic. Traditionally, the only 2 species of *Staphylococcus* recognized are:

Staphylococcus epidermidis, which is coagulase negative and nonpathogenic.

Staphylococcus aureus, which is coagulase positive and pathogenic. Recently, *Staphylococcus intermedius* and *Staphylococcus hyicus* have been added to the list of coagulase-positive pathogens. *Staphylococcus intermedius* is tube test coagulase positive, and little if any cell-bound coagulase is produced. Some strains of *Staphylococcus hyicus* produce coagulase.

Mode of Transmission

Staphylococci are extremely resistant to destruction in the environment; therefore, the organism should be considered ubiquitous (present everywhere). It is a common resident of the skin and mucous membranes, and can invade the body very easily. Staphylococcal disease is more common in areas where the organism occurs in large numbers, as in veterinary hospitals, where there are wound infections; in milking herds, where the milking machine can transmit disease; and in situations of inadequate livestock housing. An initial injury usually introduces the organism into the body to establish infection.

Pathogenicity

The pathogenicity of staphylococci is related mainly to their production of toxins, such as hemolysin, leukocidin and enterotoxin, or of enzymes, such as coagulase, hyaluronidase and penicillinase.

Staphylococcus aureus

Mastitis

This is the most common form of staphylococcal disease in cattle, sheep and goats. In recent surveys, 40% of all cases of mastitis have been associated with *Staphylococcus*. It occurs in 2 forms.

The acute form usually occurs near parturition. The infected animal shows anorexia and high fever. The infected quarter is enlarged and extremely hard, and may be gangrenous. The chronic form is characterized by small areas of induration or palpable nodules. Principal changes in the milk include clots, watery composition, increased leukocytic or somatic cell count, and increased pH.

Osteoarthritis (Bumble Foot)

This disease occurs in young birds and is characterized by subcutaneous abscesses of the foot.

Botryomycosis

This disease occurs after castration in horses. The spermatic cord becomes infected and enlarges, forming a granuloma. This infection is rare because antibiotics are commonly used for treating castration wound infections.

Otitis Externa

This is a disease of the external ear canal.

Skin and Subcutaneous Infections

These are relatively common, and may lead to abscess formation.

Urinary Infections

These typically cause straining to urinate and blood in urine.

Staphylococcus intermedius

Staphylococcus intermedius causes mastitis and pyoderma in dogs.

Staphylococcus hyicus

This organism causes polyarthritis and greasy pig disease (exudative epidermitis in swine).

Laboratory Diagnosis

Microscopic Examination: By direct examination, Gram-positive cocci can be found in stained smears of clinical specimens. The organism is rarely seen in clusters from specimens.

Culture Characteristics: The organisms grow well on common laboratory media, producing raised, shining, opaque colonies up to 4 mm in diameter. Some pathogenic species produce golden or yellow pigments. *Staphylococcus aureus* is mannitol positive and *Staph epidermidis* is mannitol negative.

Coagulase Test: This is one of the most important tests used to determine the pathogenicity of staphylococci. *Staph aureus* is coagulase positive. Several tests are used to determine if the bacterium is coagulase positive.

The coagulase tube test is the most reliable of these tests. It tests for the presence of coagulase enzyme. The coagulase slide test is a screening test for clumping factors. The Staphyloslide (BBL) and Staphaurex (Burroughs Wellcome) tests are screening tests that are more reliable than the slide test.

API Staph Identification Kit: This test (Analylab Products) differentiates among *Staphylococcus aureus, Staph intermedius* and *Staph hyicus*.

Oxidative/Fermentative Glucose (O/F) Test: This test is used to differentiate *Staphylococcus* from *Micrococcus. Staphylococcus* is fermentative, whereas *Micrococcus* is oxidative.

Treatment

Penicillinase-resistant antibiotics, such as oxicillin, cloxacillin, cephalosporin and erythromycin, are effective against *Staphylococcus* organisms. Owing to the variable susceptibility of staphylococci to antibiotics, however, antibiotic sensitivity testing should be done when possible.

Public Health Significance

Food poisoning and skin infections from staphylococci are relatively common in people.

Family: Streptococcaceae
Genus: *Streptococcus*

General Characteristics

Streptococcus organisms are Gram-positive, nonmotile cocci occurring in chains or pairs when grown in liquid media. They are aerobic, facultatively anaerobic and catalase negative. They ferment carbohydrates to produce acid but no gas. They do not form endospores.

Pathogenicity

The pathogenicity of streptococci is related mainly to their production of toxins, such as streptolysin, or enzymes, such as hyaluronidase and streptokinase.

Lancefield Groups

Streptococci are classified on the basis of their antigens. Main groups are listed below:

Lancefield

Group	Species	Disease
A	*Strep pyogenes*	Sore throat in people
B	*Strep agalactiae*	Major cause of bovine mastitis
C	*Strep dysgalactiae*	Minor cause of mastitis
	Strep equi	Strangles in horses
	Strep zooepidemicus	Genital infection, polyarthritis, wound infection
	Strep equisimilis	Infections in young pigs
D	*Strep fecalis* (Enterococci)	Urinary infection (usually a nonpathogen)
	Strep duran	Diarrhea in foals
E	*Strep suis*	Cervical lymphadenitis in pigs

Mode of Transmission

Streptococcal infection may be endogenous (from internal spread) or exogenous (of external origin). In the latter, aerosol, direct contact, fomites and ingestion are the most common sources of infection.

Streptococcus agalactiae

Streptococcus agalactiae is an obligate parasite of the mammary glands and is one of the most common causes of mastitis. It is transmitted through contaminated milkers' hands, milking machines and dairy utensils. The organism causes chronic mastitis in dairy cows. Initially the milk contains flakes. Later the milk becomes stringy and contains blood clots and purulent material. In the final stages of the disease, there are fibrosis, hardening and atrophy of the udder. Susceptibility to this disease increases with age. Acute and subacute forms of the disease are rare.

Laboratory Diagnosis

Microscopic Examination: Direct microscopic examination of milk samples reveals Gram-positive cocci in chains or pairs.

Culture Characteristics: Strep agalactiae is a fastidious organism that grows best on media containing blood or serum. On blood agar after 24 hours of incubation, the colonies are pinpoint and glistening, with beta or alpha hemolysis (Table 1).

To differentiate *Streptococcus* from *Staphylococcus,* use a catalase test. The organism is esculin negative and sodium hippurate positive.

CAMP Test: The CAMP test is used to differentiate *Streptococcus agalactiae* from other streptococci. The CAMP phenomenon is characterized by a zone of incomplete hemolysis produced by *Staphylococcus,* later becoming completely lysed by streptococcal hemolysin to produce an arrowhead appearance (Fig 1).

The CAMP test is performed as follows:

1. Streak a zone of partially hemolytic *Staph aureus* as a straight line on blood agar containing esculin.

2. Streak the suspected streptococci at a right angle to the *Staph aureus* line.

3. Incubate at 37 C for 18-24 hours until growth is evident.

4. Examine for arrowhead hemolysis (Fig 1).

5. Esculin may be incorporated into the blood agar to test for esculin hydrolysis at the same time. A positive reaction is seen as brown discoloration of the medium around the colonies.

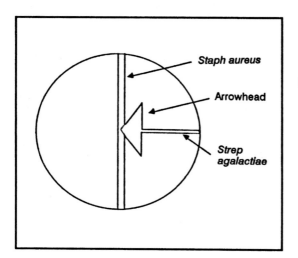

Staph aureus

Arrowhead

Strep agalactiae

Figure 1. CAMP test.

Streptococcus agalactiae is CAMP positive. *Streptococcus dysgalactiae* is CAMP negative. *Streptococcus uberis* is esculin positive and CAMP negative (Table 1).

Some laboratories use Edwards medium and examine plates under ultraviolet light (Wood's lamp). Using Edwards medium, *Strep agalactiae* forms small, transparent, bluish colonies. *Streptococcus uberis* is esculin positive, causing brown discoloration of the medium and brown colonies. *Streptococcus dysgalactiae* forms green colonies.

Streptococcus uberis

Streptococcus uberis causes mastitis, but of lesser severity than that of *Strep agalactiae*. the organism is esculin positive, producing dark brown colonies and brown discoloration of the surrounding medium (Table 1). About 10% of *Strep uberis* strains are CAMP positive, giving an arrowhead appearance.

Streptococcus dysgalactiae

Streptococcus dysgalactiae is a minor cause of mastitis. It is CAMP negative and esculin negative (Table 1).

Treatment

Streptococci are sensitive to penicillin. Intramammary infusion of mastitis preparations containing penicillin may give good results.

Control

Streptococcal infections can be controlled by: instituting good sanitation and milking procedures; detecting disease by culture methods; and treating and culturing at about 2-week intervals.

The organism can be eliminated from a dairy herd in 5 or 6 rounds of culturing and treating.

Streptococcus equi

Streptococcus equi causes strangles, which is an infection of the lymph nodes in the throat region of horses. It is more severe in young animals, as older animals seem to develop immunity.

Table 1. Differential characteristics of streptococci affecting animals.

Organism	Lance-field Group	Hemoly-sis	Tre-halose	Sorbi-tol	Manni-tol	Esculin	Lac-tose	Sodium Hippurate
Strep agalactiae	B	alpha, beta	+	–	–	–	+	+
Strep uberis		alpha, beta gamma	+	+	+	+	+	+
Strep dysgalactiae	C	alpha, gamma	+	–	–	–	+	–
Strep zooepidemicus	C	beta	–	+	–	+	+	–
Strep equi	C	beta	–	–	–	–	–	–
Strep equisimilis	C	beta	+	–	–	–	–	–
Strep canis	G	beta	–	–	–	v	+	–
Strep fecalis	D	alpha beta	+	+	+	+	+	v
Strep pyogenes	A	beta	+	–	v	+	+	–
Strep bovis	D	gamma	v	–	v	+	+	–

v = variable reaction

The incubation period is 3-6 days. Clinical signs include depression, enlargement of the mandibular lymph nodes, anorexia and fever up to 41 C. Within a few days, a serous or mucopurulent nasal discharge develops, with a dry painful, throaty cough. Within 6-21 days, the mandibular, retropharyngeal and other lymph nodes may develop draining abscesses.

Bastard strangles is a chronic form of the disease characterized by abscess formation in the internal lymph nodes. Affected horses may show signs of acute pneumonia, gastrointestinal obstruction and peritonitis.

Laboratory Diagnosis

Microscopic Examination: Direct microscopic examination of Gram-stained smears from nasal swabs and abscesses show Gram-positive cocci.

Culture Characteristics: On blood agar, *Strep equi* produces a mucoid colony with a zone of beta hemolysis (Table 1).

Treatment

Streptococcus equi is sensitive to penicillin and trimethoprim. It is controversial whether treatment with penicillin leads to bastard strangles by interfering with development of immunity. Most veterinarians agree, however, that the benefits of treatment outweigh the chance of inducing bastard strangles. Once treatment begins, it must be continued until the animal's rectal temperature remains normal for several days.

Control

Control is based on immunization, sanitation and keeping the animal from coming in contact with infected animals. Vaccination is usually not recommended unless a serious outbreak occurs, because of a problem with reaction to vaccine.

Streptococcus zooepidemicus (*Streptococcus equi* ss *zooepidemicus*)

Streptococcus zooepidemicus causes polyarthritis in young foals through infection of the umbilicus. It is also associated with infections of the cervix and uterus. *Streptococcus zooepidemicus* is the most common organism that infects the wounds of horses.

Laboratory Diagnosis

Microscopic Examination: Direct microscopic examination of a clinical specimen is used for presumptive diagnosis.

Culture Characteristics: On blood agar, *Strep zooepidemicus* produces a narrow zone of beta hemolysis (Table 1). It ferments sorbitol but not trehalose.

Streptococcus suis

This organism causes lymphadenitis of the cervical lymph nodes in swine. The mandibular lymph nodes are most frequently involved, followed by the retropharyngeal and parotid lymph nodes.

Streptococcus equisimilis

This organism causes swelling of joints in 1- to 3-week-old piglets. In the final stages, the limbs become stiff from fibrosis. Transmission is through nasal infection.

Streptococcus pneumoniae

This is primarily a human pathogen, but it also causes bronchopneumonia and meningitis in calves, and mastitis in cows.

Laboratory Diagnosis

Microscopic Examination: Direct microscopic examination reveals Gram-positive diplococci or chains.

Culture Characteristics: Colonies on blood agar are small and mucoid, and show alpha (green) hemolysis (Table 1).

Optochin Test: A specific test is for optochin sensitivity, which is 90% reliable. It is used to differentiate pneumococci from other hemolytic streptococci. In the optochin test, a disc containing optochin (DFCO) is placed on heavily inoculated blood agar and incubated at 37 C for 24 hours. *Streptococcus pneumoniae* is inhibited by optochin, whereas other streptococci are not.

Animal Inoculation: Subcutaneous injection of the organisms into mice produces rapidly developing septicemia, and death in 1-3 days.

7

Endospore-Forming Gram-Positive Bacilli

Family: Bacilliaceae
Genus: *Bacillus*
Genus: *Clostridium*
Bacillus anthracis

There are several species of the genus *Bacillus*. Most are regarded as contaminants or saprophytes. *Bacillus anthracis*, however, is of veterinary importance.

General Characteristics

Bacillus anthracis is a Gram-positive, nonmotile, aerobic, encapsulated large rod with a central spore.

Mode of Transmission

Bacillus anthracis is transmitted by inhalation of spores, ingestion of contaminated feed, and contact with infected tissue.

Pathogenicity

The pathogenicity of *Bacillus anthracis* is related to its capsule and production of toxins. The capsule tends to prevent phagocytosis. Its toxins affects the central nervous system, cardiovascular system and respiratory system.

Anthrax, the disease caused by *B anthracis*, is most common in cattle but also occurs in sheep, pigs, horses, dogs and even people. Clinical signs include fever, cardiac and respiratory distress, and a bloody discharge from body openings. In swine, the disease causes acute pharyngitis, with extensive swelling of the throat.

Laboratory Diagnosis

Direct Microscopic Examination: To protect from sporulation, the carcass of dead infected animals should never be opened. In dead affected cattle, a cut is made over the small ear vein and several smears are made directly on slides or the blood is absorbed onto a swab. In pigs, smears and swabs are taken from edematous areas in the throat. The smears are stained with methylene blue, which shows large square-ended rods with capsules. The bacteria tend to form a long chain ("box car" arrangement).

Culture Characteristics: The organism grows well on common laboratory media. Colonies appear in 24 hours and are large, glistening, mucoid, waxy at the edge, and usually nonhemolytic. If the specimen is heavily contaminated, heat it to 65 C to kill contaminant organisms and then streak it. This organism should not be cultured except by reference laboratories.

Treatment

Penicillin with streptomycin is recommended in the early stages of anthrax. Oxytetracycline and chlortetracycline are the antibiotics of choice.

Control

Because anthrax is transmissible to people, personnel working with anthrax outbreaks must be extremely careful. They should use rubber suits, rubber gloves and rubber shoes that are sterilized before leaving the premises. If an infected animal is admitted to a veterinary hospital, it is necessary to completely disinfect the entire premises with strong concentrated lye.

Never open the carcass of an animal thought to have died from anthrax, as large numbers of organisms are present in the blood and tissues. On exposure to air, the organisms could sporulate. Notify your state animal health authorities immediately. Spores of *B anthracis* can live in soil for almost 40 years; therefore, the carcass should be burned or disposed of by deep burial.

Clostridium Species

General Characteristics

Clostridium is a large motile, anaerobic, nonencapsulated, catalase-negative, spore-forming, Gram-positive rod with rounded ends. Spores may vary in their shape, size and location in the bacterial cell (Fig 1).

Based on invasiveness, clostridia can be divided into 2 groups:

Invasive Group: This group invades and multiplies in tissues and also produces toxins. Included in this group are *Clostridium chauveoi, Cl septicum, Cl novyi* and *Cl perfringens*. These organisms cause a number of diseases, including blackleg and malignant edema, in large and small animals, and have been isolated form wounds, fractures and surgical incisions.

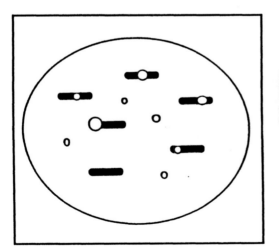

Figure 1. Clostridial spores vary in their size, shape and location in the bacterial cell. In this illustration, some have escaped from the bacterial cells.

Noninvasive Group: This group does not invade tissues and produces disease by production of very potent toxins. This group includes *Clostridium tetani* and *Cl botulinum*.

Clostridium chauvoei

This organism causes blackleg in young ruminants 4 months to 2 years of age. The initial signs are fever and lameness, followed by swelling over the region of heavy muscles. Gas produced in tissues causes a crackling sound on palpation (crepitation) like crumpling newspaper. Lesions consist of blackened muscular tissue at the site of the swelling. Affected sheep have a stiff gait and severe lameness but no skin crepitation. Mortality is nearly 100%. Blackleg causes serious economic losses.

Mode of Transmission

The organism is present in the soil and in the gastrointestinal tract of herbivores. It is usually transmitted by ingestion or through wounds, such as from castration or dehorning. The peak incidence is usually in the summer.

Clostridium septicum

This organism is similar to *Clostridium chauvoei* in general characteristics and causes malignant edema in cattle, sheep, horses and pigs. Lesions are characterized by extensive tissue swelling that is soft and cold, and pits on pressure. Affected animals are stiff and lame. Death occurs within 24-48 hours.

Clostridium hemolyticum

This organism causes bacillary hemoglobinuria or red water disease in cattle. This disease is characterized by anemia, high fever, abdominal pain, an enlarged liver, bile-stained feces and dark red urine. The disease is prevalent in liver fluke-infested areas, and liver flukes are thought to predispose to the disease.

Mode of Transmission

This disease occurs in low-lying swampy areas in summer. Ingestion of contaminated feed is the main route of infection.

Clostridium novyi

The most common disease caused by this organism is black disease, which is associated with migrating liver flukes. Clinical signs include abdominal pain, rapid shallow breathing, cold skin and reluctance to move. On necropsy, the liver is enlarged and the inner surface of the skin is darkened by blood-stained edema; hence the name "black disease."

Clostridium perfringens

This organism produces multiple syndromes based on the type of toxin produced.

Cl perfringens Type A: This is the most widespread type and causes hemorrhagic gastroenteritis in dogs.

Cl perfringens Type B: This type causes dysentery in lambs during the first 2 weeks of life.

Cl perfringens Type C: This type causes hemorrhagic enteritis in neonatal calves and piglets.

Cl perfringens Type D: This type causes "overeating disease," a disease of feedlot sheep that is most common in North America. When animals are given high-grain rations, the large amount of grain provides an ideal growth medium for the organism. The animals absorb the toxin and may die quickly. It is also called pulpy kidney disease because the kidneys become enlarged and decomposed.

Laboratory Diagnosis of Clostridial Disease

Microscopic Examination: Direct microscopic examination of tissue specimens with Gram stain is often helpful. Specimens should be obtained soon after death. Fluorescent antibody testing is the test of choice for *Cl chauveoi, Cl septicum* and *Cl novyi* infection.

Culture Characteristics: Culture of clostridial organisms is difficult and will not be discussed in this text.

Animal Inoculation: Mouse and guinea pig inoculation is the most common test used to diagnose *Cl perfringens* and *Cl hemolyticum* infections.

Treatment

Penicillin, tetracycline and chloramphenicol are useful in clostridial infections.

Control

Vaccination is the best method of control. Numerous multivalent vaccines are available. Good hygiene at calving, lambing, docking, shearing and castrating is also important. Carcasses of animals that have died of clostridial infection should be burned or buried to prevent soil contamination.

Clostridium tetani

Clostridium tetani affects mainly horses and people, but other animals can also become infected. The organism produces a neurotoxin that causes the disease called tetanus or lockjaw. The most common signs are loss of appetite, erect ears, tail held out stiffly and general stiffness giving the appearance of a sawhorse stance. Prolapse of the third eyelid and muscular spasms also are apparent. Animals may go into violent convulsions upon hearing a sudden noise.. Hyperesthesia, which is an exaggerated response to normal stimulus, may be apparent. Because of paralysis of the masseter muscles, the animal is unable to open its mouth; hence the term lockjaw. Death is from respiratory failure.

Mode of Transmission

The organism is widespread throughout the world. It is found in the soil and in intestines. The infectious agent is transmitted through a puncture wound.

Laboratory Diagnosis

Microscopic Examination: Clinical signs of tetanus are so characteristic that it is seldom confused with other diseases. When specimens are obtained, microscopic examination shows Gram-positive rods with terminal swollen spores that give the appearance of a tennis racket (Fig 1).

Animal Inoculation: Mouse inoculation may be used to demonstrate the presence of toxins.

Therapy and Control

Penicillin combined with antitoxin is useful in treatment of tetanus. If a wound is found, treat it locally and drain. Muscle relaxants may help prevent muscle twitching. Immunization is provided with tetanus toxoid, which is sometimes combined with influenza and sleeping sickness vaccine. Tetanus toxoid and antitoxin should be given after castration, tail docking and traumatic wounds.

Public Health Significance

Clostridium tetani is transmissible to people through puncture wounds.

Clostridium botulinum

Clostridium botulinum causes botulism through ingestion of food contaminated with the organism, which elaborates potent neurotoxins. The organism produces a number of distinct types of toxins, classified as A, B, C, D, E and F. Only types A, B, C and D are of veterinary importance.

Type A causes progressive muscular paralysis, particularly of the jaw and throat. Affected animals become recumbent and die of respiratory failure.

Type B causes shaker foal syndrome. Affected foals can stand when assisted but then begin to shake and drop to the ground.

Type C causes "limberneck" in ducks and wild birds. Affected birds show paralysis of the wings, legs and neck, and cannot retract the nictitating membrane.

Type D affects cattle in South Africa in certain restricted areas on the range. The disease is associated with phosphorus deficiency and is called Lamziekte or lame sickness.

Laboratory Diagnosis

Mouse inoculation is used to demonstrate the presence of the toxin in the serum.

Treatment

Early use of specific antitoxic serum and a purgative to remove toxins may be helpful.

8

Gram-Positive
Non-Spore-Forming Bacilli

Listeria Species

General Characteristics

Members of this genus are small Gram-positive pleomorphic rods. They are catalase positive, aerobic, and motile with tumbling motility at room temperature. On blood agar colonies are small, blue and pinpoint sized, like streptococci, with a narrow zone of beta hemolysis. Stab cultures on semisolid motility media produce a typical inverted pine tree formation. It does not liquefy gelatin, and growth is favored by addition of glucose.

Mode of Transmission

These organisms are found in soil, feces, genital secretions and moldy hay. The mode of transmission is not precisely known. Listeriosis in farm animals is associated with feeding silage, particularly corn silage, and occurs in colder climates.

Listeria monocytogenes

The organism causes listeriosis or circling disease in ruminants. The disease affects animals of all ages and is characterized by meningoencephalitis. In the early stages, the animal crowds into a corner and walks in a circle, usually in one direction. The neck is stiff, with the head held to one side. Finally there is paralysis of the limbs. Abortions may occur in cows and ewes with no other signs of disease. An acute septicemic form is common in young monogastric animals, particularly in foals. It is characterized by depression, emaciation and dyspnea.

Laboratory Diagnosis

Microscopic Examination: Though the organism localizes in the medulla and pons, it is often difficult to recover. Gram stains and fluorescent antibody testing of tissue imprints are useful.

Culture Characteristics: Ground brain is stored at refrigerator temperature and cultured weekly for up to 8 weeks before proclaiming a negative result.

Animal Inoculation: Intracerebral inoculation of mice may accelerate confirmation of the diagnosis.

Treatment

Tetracycline in large doses appears to give good results, but treatment is usually of no value after central nervous system signs appear.

Public Health Significance

This disease is transmissible to people. Owners, veterinarians and veterinary technicians should be careful when handling materials associated with abortions. Organisms are secreted in milk, and consumption of infected milk and chewing moldy hay have caused the disease in people.

Erysipelothrix Species

General Characteristics

Members of this genus are small, slim, Gram-positive rods. Curved filamentous forms also are seen. The organism is nonmotile, nonspore forming, catalase negative and aerobic. It grows on common laboratory media. The colonies initially are smooth and glistening buttons 1 mm in diameter that, after 48 hours, become opaque to gray. Stab cultures on semisolid media produce a test tube brush appearance. The organism is alpha hemolytic.

Mode of Transmission

Ingestion of contaminated feed or water is considered to be the source of infection. Houseflies and ticks may carry the organism. The disease is more common in the summer due to high temperatures and fluctuations in environmental temperature. Healthy carrier animals may exist.

Erysipelothrix rhusiopathiae

This organism is mainly associated with swine and causes erysipelas. It can also cause disease in other animals. Erysipelas in swine occurs in 3 forms:

Acute Septicemia: The onset is sudden, with prostration, high fever, walking on the toes, and sudden death. This form commonly occurs in suckling pigs.

Skin Form (Diamond Skin Disease): Affected pigs have diamond-shaped plaques of variable size and number on the skin of the abdomen, ears and snout. The skin may slough in severely affected animals.

Chronic Form: This form is a sequel to the acute form. Chronically affected animals develop endocarditis and/or polyarthritis.

Laboratory Diagnosis

Microscopic Examination: Direct microscopic examination of Gram-stained smears of skin lesions or the spleen of a dead animal shows Gram-positive rods. The colonies are alpha hemolytic, oxidase negative and nonmotile.

Culture Characteristics: Table 1 lists the criteria used to differentiate this organism from streptococci, which are also catalase negative, and *Listeria*, which closely resembles this organism.

Treatment

Hyperimmune serum should be given early in the disease. Penicillin therapy also yields good results.

Table 1. Characteristics used to differentiate *Listeria*, *Erysipelothrix* and *Streptococcus*.

	Listeria monocytogenes	L rhusiopathiae	Streptococcus
Morphology	Small Rod	Slim rod	Cocci
Catalase test	Positive	Negative	Negative
Motility	Motile (tumbling)	Nonmotile	Nonmotile
TSI (H_2S)	Negative	Positive	Negative
Test tube brush appearance in gelatin	No	Yes	No

Control

Control is based upon immunization. Sanitation alone will not eliminate the disease. Sows and piglets should be immunized with the various bacterins and modified-live vaccines available.

Public Health Significance

This organism is transmissible to people and causes a skin disease called erysipeloid. The lesions are usually found on the hands. The portal of entry is a skin wound. Veterinary technicians should be extra careful when handling the modified-live vaccine or hogs showing signs of erysipelas.

9

Gram-Negative Facultatively Anaerobic Bacilli

Family: Enterobacteriaceae

General Characteristics

Members of this family are small Gram-negative rods or coccobacilli. They can be motile or nonmotile, aerobic or facultatively anaerobic, catalase positive and oxidase negative. Acid is produced by fermentation of glucose and other carbohydrates by several genera.

Mode of Transmission

Most members of this family are part of the normal flora of the intestine but can become pathogens under certain circumstances. Navel infections and ingestion of contaminated feces are the main portals of entry of these organisms. Some important members of this family are *Escherichia coli*, *Salmonella arizona*, *Klebsiella* and *Proteus*.

Escherichia coli

Escherichia coli organisms are small Gram-negative rods or coccobacilli that are motile by means of peritrichous flagella. They are aerobic or facultatively anaerobic, ferment lactose with gas production, and produce indole. The organism grows well on nutrient agar at 37 C. Colonies may be smooth or rough. Smooth colonies are low, convex, gray or colorless, moist and shiny. Rough colonies have a dry appearance and do not emulsify easily in water.

The organisms have 3 surface antigens called O (somatic), K (capsular) and H (flagellar). On MacConkey agar, coliform organisms produce deep red colonies because of fermentation of lactose. *Escherichia coli* is indole positive and produces acid and gas from glucose, lactose and sucrose. On triple sugar iron (TSI), it produces an acid slant, acid butt, and usually gas. *Escherichia coli* is responsible for many neonatal infections in calves, swine, sheep and puppies.

Infectious Colibacillosis of Calves: *Escherichia coli* is an opportunist and is especially virulent in neonatal calves that are stressed or lack immunity to pathogens because of little or no transfer of immunoglobulins from the dam.

Calf Scours: Calf scours is one of the most common syndromes caused by *E coli* K-99. It is most prevalent in North America and usually occurs in animals less than 2 weeks old. Predisposing factors include lack of colostrum intake, cold wet conditions, and overcrowding. Diarrhea is the main sign. The feces are profuse, liquid and yellow or gray. Dehydration and loss of electrolytes may result in death.

Colibacillosis of Piglets: Piglet scours is caused by *E coli* K-88 strain. Piglets develop diarrhea during the first few hours or days of life and become dehydrated. They do not refuse to nurse, but they vomit, as in transmissible gastroenteritis. The intestines are distended with gas and mucus. The cause of death is dehydration and electrolyte imbalance.

Colibacillosis of Weanling Pigs: This is a disease of weaned pigs, usually 8-12 weeks old. Affected pigs are usually found dead. There is edema of the eyelids, forehead, ears, elbow and hock joints. Such neurologic signs as muscular incoordination and partial hind leg paralysis may be seen.

Colibacillosis of Lambs: This disease occurs in 2 forms. The septic form is more common and is usually found in 2- to 3-week-old lambs. Acutely infected lambs show septicemia and sudden collapse. Neurologic signs are also noted. The enteric form is similar to calf scours.

Mastitis: Mastitis due to *E coli* has become a serious problem in recent years. This may be attributed to the growing size of dairy herds kept in close confinement during winter months, and to extensive treatment programs for elimination of other udder pathogens.

Laboratory Diagnosis

Culture Characteristics: *Escherichia coli* can be isolated from the feces using the protocol outlined in Table 1. The strain of *E coli* causing calf scours has the K-99 antigen, while that causing piglet scours has the K-88 antigen. Using the fluorescent antibody technique, *E coli* strains K-99 and K-88 appear apple green when viewed with a microscope equipped with ultraviolet light. Table 2 lists the criteria for biochemical identification of *E coli*.

Treatment

Except for colibacillosis in weanling pigs, other cases of colibacillosis are treated with broad-spectrum antibacterials, such as ampicillin, trimethoprim and chloramphenicol, and fluid therapy.

Control

Colibacillosis can be controlled by ensuring good colostrum intake during the first few hours of life, providing proper housing and good hygiene, and vaccinating susceptible animals.

Salmonella Species

Salmonella is a Gram-negative rod that is motile by peritrichous flagella (except *S gallinarum* and *S pullorum*). Most strains do not ferment lactose or sucrose (except *S arizonae*). The organism is aerobic or facultatively anaerobic.

Table 1. Protocol for identification of Enterobacteriaceae.

1. Plate the fecal sample on blood agar and MacConkey agar.
2. For *Salmonella*, inoculate tetrathionate broth/selenite broth and brilliant green agar.
3. For *Salmonella* subculture, plate on MacConkey agar and on brilliant green, if necessary. *Salmonella* serotyping must be done at a reference lab.
4. Inoculate TSI, citrate, indole, Hektoen and methyl red for conventional biochemical tests (Table 3).
5. Confirm identification using API or Enterotube.

Table 2. Criteria for identification of Enterobacteriaceae.

Medium	Lactose Fermenters			Nonlactose Fermenters	
	E coli	Klebsiella	Enterobacter	Proteus	Salmonella Species
MacConkey agar	Red	Light pink, mucoid	Red	Colorless	Colorless
Brilliant green agar	Yellow-green	Yellow-green	Yellow-green	Red	Red
TSI slant	Yellow	Yellow	Yellow	Red	Red
TSI butt	Yellow with gas	Yellow with gas	Yellow with gas	Yellow with gas & H_2S	Yellow with gas & H_2S
Urea	−	+	−	+	−
Citrate	−	+	+	±	±
Indole	+	−	−	±	±
Motility	+	−	+	+	+
Hektoen agar	Orange-red	Orange-red	Orange-red	Blue-Green l H_2S	Blue-green ± with H_2S
Methyl red	+	−	−	−	−
Lactose broth	Yellow with gas	Yellow with gas	Yellow with or without gas	−	−
S.S. agar	Somewhat inhibited, red-pink	Not mucoid, red-pink	Red-pink	Colorless with black center	Colorless with or without black center
Bismuth sulfite	Usually inhibited, green or brown	Usually inhibited, green or brown	Usually inhibited, green or brown	Usually inhibited, green or brown	Black rabbit eye

On the basis of host susceptibility, *Salmonella* species may be divided into 3 groups. Human pathogens affect only people and include *S typhi* and *S paratyphi*. Primarily animal pathogens may also affect people but primarily affect animals. These include *S typhimurium* and *S dublin*. Animal pathogens affect only animals, and include *S pullorum*, *S gallinarum*, *S abortus equi* and *S abortus ovis*.

Forms of *Salmonella* Infection

There are 2 forms of *Salmonella* infections in animals.

Septic Form: Young animals are the most susceptible. In this form, there is generally no diarrhea. The animal has a high fever and increased respiration and pulse, accompanied by neurologic signs. Mortality is very high, approaching 100%.

Enteric Form: Acute enteritis is more common in older animals and is characterized by severe watery diarrhea, high fever and rapid pulse and respiratory rates. The feces have a putrid odor and may contain mucus and casts. Chronic enteritis is more common in older animals and is characterized by persistent diarrhea, severe emaciation and intermittent fever. The feces may be blood tinged and contain mucus. Food poisoning from *Salmonella* is seen in people but not in animals.

Salmonella species responsible for infection in cattle are *S dublin* and *S typhimurium*. Neonatal calves are affected by the septicemic form, whereas calves more than a week old are affected by the enteric form. Pregnant cows may abort. After recovery, cows serve as carriers of the disease.

Salmonella abortus equi is the most common cause of salmonellosis in horses. In foals, it causes navel infections, septicemia and/or polyarthritis. Mares may abort in later stages.

Salmonella typhimurium and *S newport* may cause acute enteritis following stress, such as from transport, surgery or administration of an anthelmintic.

Two species of *Salmonella* cause disease in poultry. *Salmonella pullorum* causes mild diarrhea with white feces. *Salmonella gallinarum* causes greenish diarrhea. Poultry serve as the main reservoir for *Salmonella*.

Salmonella typhimurium causes acute septicemia and gastroenteritis in cats and dogs, particularly in puppies and kittens or animals crowded in unsanitary conditions.

Swine are another reservoir of *Salmonella*. The main species in swine are *S typhimurium* and *S dublin*. These cause enteritis, septicemia and pneumonia.

Laboratory Diagnosis

Culture Characteristics: *Salmonella* can usually be isolated from clinical specimens with relative ease on ordinary lab media (Table 2). Colonies may be smooth or rough. Smooth colonies have a glossy surface with a regular edge, whereas rough colonies are granular with an irregular edge.

Salmonella does not ferment lactose and produces pale to colorless colonies on MacConkey agar, bright pink colonies on brilliant green agar, and blue-green colonies with black centers and H_2S production on Hektoen agar. It is indole negative, urease negative and citrate positive (Table 2).

Treatment

Ampicillin, trimethroprim, tetracycline and chloramphenicol are usually effective against *Salmonella* infections.

Klebsiella Species

The general characteristics of this genus are similar to those of *E coli*, except *Klebsiella* is nonmotile and usually has a capsule. On culture media, colonies are mucoid. *Klebsiella* causes bovine mastitis that is indistinguishable from *E coli* mastitis. In horses it causes metritis and abortion.

Laboratory Diagnosis

Culture Characteristics: On ordinary media, growth is mucoid. *Klebsiella* ferments lactose with gas production (Table 2). *Klebsiella* is citrate and urease positive.

Treatment

The most useful antibiotics against *Klebsiella* are erythromycin, gentamicin and neomycin.

Arizona Species

Organisms in this genus cause diarrhea in turkeys.

Proteus Species

Some species of *Proteus* produce a unique swarming growth on regular laboratory media. On cystine lactose electrolyte-deficient (CLED) media or those containing 6% agar or sulfadiazone, this effect is not produced. It is urease positive, nonlactose fermenting and H_2S positive, and produces colorless colonies on MacConkey agar (Table 2). *Proteus* species produce a distinctive putrid odor on culture.

Family: Pasteurellaceae
Genus: *Pasteurella*

General Characteristics

Members of this genus are small Gram-negative coccobacilli or rods showing bipolar staining. The organisms are aerobic, facultatively anaerobic, and catalase and oxidase positive. Some produce an indole-positive reaction. Only 2 species of *Pasteurella* are of importance in veterinary medicine.

Pasteurella hemolytica

Pasteurella hemolytica is the principal agent involved in pneumonic pasteurellosis or shipping fever; however, *P multocida* and other bacteria and viruses may also cause pneumonia. The disease usually follows such stress as transport, dehorning, castration, weaning, adverse weather and starvation. The disease is characterized by high fever, anorexia, dyspnea, coughing, nasal discharge and pneumonia.

Some cases in any group of newly arrived weaned feeder calves are inevitable. Cattle of any age can be affected, but animals 2-6 years old are more susceptible. The incidence of *P hemolytica* infection is greatest during the autumn due to the movement of cattle and sudden changes in the weather.

Mode of Transmission

Direct contact and aerosol inhalation are main routes of infection.

Laboratory Diagnosis

Microscopic Examination: Direct microscopic examination of clinical specimens reveals Gram-negative ellipsoid rods with uniform staining.

Culture Characteristics: On blood agar, the colonies vary from smooth to mucoid and rough. *Pasteurella hemolytica* produces a narrow zone of beta hemolysis. Table 3 lists the criteria used to differentiate between *Pasteurella hemolytica* and *Pasteurella multocida.*

Treatment

Such antibacterial drugs as sulfamethazine and oxytetracycline are commonly used.

Prevention and Control

Infection by *P hemolytica* is controlled in a number of ways. Minimizing stress is helpful but not easy. The main stress factors are castration, dehorning, weaning and shipping. Preconditioning programs are also useful. These are certified feeder cattle programs involving feeding, weaning, vaccination and parasite control. The animals are identified by green ear tags applied by a veterinarian and accompanied by a certificate. The efficacy of these programs has been questioned.

Preimmunization programs include all preconditioning techniques, except that the calves are not weaned and are identified by *white* ear tags applied by the veterinarian and accompanied by a certificate.

Prophylactic drugs should be given after shipment of cattle. Early identification of sick animals and thorough prompt aggressive treatment are crucial to minimize losses. New members of a herd should be isolated to confine the disease. Animals should be gradually introduced to concentrates to allow them to adjust to dietary changes. Finally, good ventilation and appropriate vaccinations help reduce infection.

Table 3. Criteria used to differentiate *Pasteurella multocida* from *P hemolytica*.

	Pasteurella multocida	Pasteurella hemolytica
Indole	+	–
MacConkey agar	No growth	Small pink colonies
Blood agar	No hemolysis	Beta hemolysis
In case of doubt, identify with the API system.		

Pasteurella multocida

This organism produces a wide variety of diseases in animals. In cattle, *P multocida* produces pneumonia that may vary from an acute to chronic infection. *Pasteurella multocida* is part of the normal flora in the mouth of dogs and cats. It occurs as a secondary invader in wounds caused by biting.

In poultry, *P multocida* causes fowl cholera, characterized by acute enteritis, chronic arthritis and wound infection. In rabbits, *P multocida* causes snuffles, characterized by pneumonia and upper respiratory infections. *Pasteurella multocida* causes swine plague, usually as a complication of viral pneumonia.

Laboratory Diagnosis

Culture Characteristics: There is no growth on MacConkey agar. On blood agar, colonies are of moderate size and non-hemolytic, and have a sweetish or musty odor.

Hemophilus Species

General Characteristics

Members of this genus are small, nonmotile, microaerophilic (require CO_2), facultatively anaerobic Gram-negative rods or coccobacilli that require hemin and nicotinamide-adenine-dinucleotide (NAD), commonly referred to as X and V factors, respectively.

Transmission

The mechanism of transmission is not precisely known. The organism is commensal on the mucous membranes of the respiratory tract and occasionally the genital tract, and an aerosol route has been suggested. Shipping stress, changes in climate, and crowding predispose animals to *Hemophilus* infection.

Hemophilus somnus

Hemophilus somnus causes a classic disease of feedlot cattle called infectious thromboembolic meningoencephalitis. It occurs in the fall, usually a few weeks after arrival in feedlots and is characterized in the early stages by reluctance to move and a staggering gait. Affected animals have a fever as high as 42 C and hemorrhages in the retina. The animal may respond to antibiotic treatment at this stage. If neurologic signs develop, the disease is too advanced for treatment. Major neurologic signs include stupor, opisthotonus, ataxia and paralysis. At necropsy, the most important findings are single or multiple hemorrhagic foci in the brain.

Other clinical infections associated with *Hemophilus somnus* are pneumonia, arthritis, and genital infections.

Hemophilus suis and *H parasuis*

These organisms cause Glasser's disease in young pigs, characterized by fever, anorexia, depression, dyspnea and polyarthritis. This infection is more common in Europe.

Actinobacillus (Hemophilus) pleuropneumoniae

This organism causes pleuropneumonia and septicemia in swine, the most common infection of swine in Canada.

Hemophilus gallinarum

This organism causes fowl coryza, characterized by nasal discharge, sneezing and facial swelling.

Taylorella (Hemophilus) equigenitalis

This organism causes a highly contagious venereal infection known as contagious equine metritis of equidae. The disease is characterized by a profuse grayish-white, sticky mucopurulent vulvar discharge lasting 2 weeks. Fertility is decreased. Infected stallions show no clinical signs and are carriers.

Laboratory Diagnosis

Culture Characteristics: *Hemophilus* is a fastidious organism that requires X and/or V factors for growth (Table 4). Blood contains X factor, while *Staph aureus* supplies V factor. Discs impregnated with these factors are also available commercially. When the organism is inoculated onto blood agar with a *Staph*

Table 4. Characteristics of *Hemophilus* species.

Species	Species Affected	Factors Required		Disease
		X*	V**	
H somnus	Cattle	+	–	Thromboembolic encephalomeningitis
H suis	Swine	+	+	Glasser's disease
H gallinarum	Chickens	+	+	Infectious coryza
Taylorella (*Hemophilus*) *equigenitalis*	Horses	+	–	Contagious equine metritis

x* = hemin
v** = nicotinamide adenine dinucleotide (NAD)

streak or disc impregnated with V factor, small translucent, circular satellite colonies appear adjacent to the *Staph* streak or the disc (Fig 1).

The organism grows best in a 5-10% CO_2 atmosphere. Chocolate agar contains X and V factor and is used more commonly. Colonies on this agar are larger and opalescent. The organism does not produce satellite colonies on chocolate agar.

Treatment

Oxytetracycline and sulfonamides are effective against *Hemophilus* species.

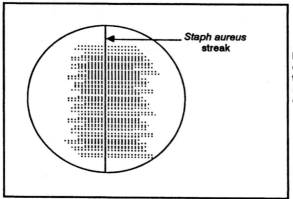

Staph aureus streak

Figure 1. *Hemophilus suis* colonies growing adjacent to a streak of *Staph aureus* (satellite growth) on a plate of blood agar.

Actinobacillus Species

General Characteristics

These organisms are small Gram-negative rods. Both pleomorphic and filamentous forms occur. They are facultative
anerobes that ferment lactose and/or sucrose (Table 5). Colony
morphology is similar to that of *Pasteurella*. They are indole
negative, trehalose negative and urease positive, and produce
H_2S.

Mode of Transmission

These organisms are present in the oral cavity of healthy
animals. Infection is established after oral trauma.

Actinobacillus lignieresii

This organism produces wooden tongue in cattle. It affects
areas of the head, such as the tongue, pharynx and hard palate.
Granulomatous lesions contain foci of greenish pus.

Laboratory Diagnosis

Microscopic Examination: When pus or granular material is
placed in a Petri plate and washed with distilled water, the
gray-white granules can be seen with a hand lens or under low
power of the microscope.

Culture Characteristics: The organism grows well on blood
agar in a 10% CO_2 atmosphere. The colonies are small, bluish,
smooth and glistening.

Table 5. Criteria for differentiating *Actinobacillus* species.

Species	Gelatin Liquefaction	Urease	Fermentation	
			Lactose	Sucrose
A lignieresii	–	+	+	+
A equuli	+	+	+	+
A suis	–	+	+	+
Pasteurella hemolytica	–	–	+	·+

Treatment

Wooden tongue lesions can be treated by swabbing iodine on the lesion. Sodium iodide can be administered IV or potassium iodide can be administered orally. Oral sulfonamides and systemic tetracycline also are effective.

Actinobacillus equuli

Actinobacillus equuli causes septicemia and purulent infections of joints and kidneys. The disease is frequently called shigellosis, which is incorrect. Foals become infected at birth through navel infections.

Laboratory Diagnosis

Culture Characteristics: This organism grows well on blood agar. The colonies are rough and mucoid.

Treatment

Streptomycin, chlortetracycline and chloramphenicol give good results.

Control

Actinobacillus equuli infections are prevented with good sanitation at parturition. Infected mares should be culled or treated.

10

Gram-Negative Aerobic Bacilli

Family: Pseudomonadaceae
Genus: *Pseudomonas*

General Characteristics

Pseudomonas organisms are Gram-negative, nonspore-form-ing, strictly aerobic, slightly curved or straight rods. They are motile, catalase positive, oxidase positive and indole negative, and do not ferment sugars (Table 1).

Pathogenicity

The organism produces hemolysin, lecithinase, protease and leukocidin, all of which play a role in the production of disease.

Mode of Transmission

Pseudomonas is a common inhabitant of the soil and the nasal cavity. It is frequently found as a contaminant of surgical wounds, utensils and equipment.

Pseudomonas aeruginosa

Pseudomonas aeruginosa causes urinary and ear infections in dogs, eye and reproductive problems in horses, mastitis, traumatic pericarditis and abortion in cattle, necrotic rhinitis and pneumonia in swine, enzootic pneumonia in mink and chinchilla, and green wool disease in sheep.

Laboratory Diagnosis

Microscopic Examination: Stained smears from a clinical specimen (usually green pus) show Gram-negative cigar-shaped rods that are difficult to differentiate morphologically from enteric bacteria.

Culture Characteristics: The organism commonly produces blue-green pigments with a fruity odor, characteristic of the species. It liquefies gelatin and turns litmus milk a watery deep blue. It produces growth on MacConkey agar. It produces an oxidative reaction on the O/F test, and alkaline reactions on the TSI slants. Table 1 lists reactions used to differentiate *Pseudomonas* from *Aeromonas* and Enterobacteriaceae.

Treatment

Pseudomonas infections are difficult to treat. Such antibiotics as polymixin B locally and gentamicin systemically are useful.

Brucella Species

General Characteristics

These organisms are Gram-negative, nonmotile, nonspore-forming small rods or coccobacilli that are microaerophilic, and catalase and urease positive. They require CO_2 for culturing (especially *B abortus*).

Mode of Transmission

The oral route is the most common route of infection. Venereal and skin routes are less common. The important species of *Brucella* are *B abortus*, *B melitensis*, *B suis* and *B canis*.

Table 1. Reactions used to differentiate *Pseudomonas* from *Aeromonas* and Enterobacteriaceae.

Test	Pseudomonas	Aeromonas	Enterobacteriaceae
Oxidase	+	+	−
O/F	Oxidative	Fermentative	Oxidative/fermentative

Brucella abortus

Brucella abortus causes brucellosis or Bang's disease, characterized by abortion at 5-6 months of pregnancy in cattle. Retained fetal membranes and metritis are common complications. In cows, the infection localizes in the gravid uterus, udder and spleen. After abortion, cows act as carriers through their milk and vaginal mucus. In bulls, occasionally the infection localizes in the testicles, epididymis or seminal vesicle, and forms abscesses. Brucellosis is a disease of great economic importance. Many countries spend millions of dollars to eradicate it.

Laboratory Diagnosis

Microscopic Examination: Modified acid-fast stain is useful to demonstrate *Brucella* in smears from clinical specimens, such as stomach contents of the aborted fetus and fetal fluids.

Culture Characteristics: *Brucella* requires a 10% CO_2 atmosphere for culture. The organism grows slowly and requires 3-5 days of incubation. The organism is transmitted to people and is potentially dangerous to work with. Send samples to a reference laboratory for isolation and identification. Serologic tests are common, but false-positive or false-negative tests may occur.

Serologic Examination: The test is based on the presence of antibodies against the *Brucella* organism. The Brewer card test is one of the most common screening tests for brucellosis. For confirmation, send samples to a reference laboratory for a tube agglutination test.

Control

Canada is free of brucellosis, as are many states in the United States. A modified-live vaccine, strain 19, is about 70% effective.

Public Health Significance

Brucella abortus organisms are an occupational hazard for veterinarians, farmers, butchers and veterinary technicians. They cause undulant fever in people. People should use caution when handling aborted fetuses.

Brucella ovis causes infertility in rams due to epididymitis. Adult rams are affected more commonly.

Brucella melitensis

Brucella melitensis causes abortion in goats.

Brucella canis

Brucella canis causes lymphadenitis, abortion and testicular atrophy in dogs. A slide agglutination test kit is available (Pitman-Moore) to diagnose canine *Brucella* infection.

Bordetella Species

General Characteristics

Bordetella organisms are small, Gram-negative rods and coccobacilli that are motile by peritrichous flagella. They are oxidase, urease, citrate and indole negative. They do not ferment carbohydrates, and turn litmus milk markedly alkaline.

Mode of Transmission

The organism is commensal in the upper respiratory tract of dogs and swine, and is often a secondary invader in dogs with distemper. It may be endogenous and spread by droplet inhalation.

Bordetella bronchiseptica

Bordetella bronchiseptica is a cause of kennel cough or bronchopneumonia in dogs, and may be associated with canine distemper. The disease is characterized by tracheobronchitis, exercise intolerance, and a honking, nonproductive cough. In swine, *B bronchiseptica* causes atrophic rhinitis. Usually young animals 3-8 weeks old are affected. It affects the turbinate bones, resulting in upward or lateral deviation of the nose.

Laboratory Diagnosis

Culture Characteristics: On blood agar, colonies are small and dewdrop-like. MacConkey agar gives grayish-tan colonies.

Treatment

Sulfonamides and broad-spectrum antibiotics are useful.

Francisella Species

General Characteristics

Members of the *Francisella* genus are very small, pleomorphic coccoid, Gram-negative and microaerophilic, and require CO_2 for growth. No growth develops on ordinary medium. A medium containing cystine, such as egg yolk or blood-glucose-cystine agar, is necessary for growth. They produce acid and no gas in glucose, maltose and mannitol.

Mode of Transmission

Infection is transmitted by the bite of infected wood ticks, *Dermacentor andersoni,* and ingestion of contaminated feed and water.

Francisella tularensis

Francisella tularensis causes tularemia in sheep, rabbits and other wild mammals. It is characterized by fever and elevated respiratory rates. Affected sheep show diarrhea, coughing, lymphadenitis and loss of wool.

Laboratory Diagnosis

Culture Characteristics: The organism grows well on blood-dextrose-cystine agar.

Serologic Examination: The agglutination test is used in serologic diagnosis.

Animal Inoculation: Guinea pig and mice inoculation is satisfactory.

Treatment

Streptomycin and tetracycline are effective.

Control

Sheep should be kept away from contaminated pastures. Efforts should be made to control the tick and rodent population. Ingestion of contaminated food and water should be prevented.

Public Health Significance

People are infected by handling infected wildlife, such as rabbits, rodents and deer, or from eating incompletely cooked meat and drinking contaminated water.

11

Gram-Negative Cocci or Coccobacilli

Family: Neisseriaceae
Genus: *Moraxella*

General Characteristics

Moraxella organisms are small Gram-negative diplobacilli or diplococci that are nonmotile, aerobic, and catalase and oxidase positive. They do not ferment carbohydrates, and slowly liquefy gelatin.

Moraxella bovis

This is the only species of importance in veterinary medicine. The organism causes infectious bovine keratoconjunctivitis (IBK) or pinkeye. The initial sign is a serous ocular discharge that later becomes mucopurulent. Other signs are slight cloudiness of the cornea, bloodshot eyes, squinting and photophobia. In the chronic form, corneal ulceration develops. This disease affects a large number of animals in a herd.

Mode of Transmission

Solar radiation predisposes cattle to pinkeye. It is more common in the summer, just after periods of peak solar radiation. White-faced cattle are more susceptible. Black-faced cattle or cattle with black pigment around the eyes seldom get the disease. Flies carry infectious ocular discharge from one animal to another. Cows rubbing each other or other objects also transmit the disease.

Laboratory Diagnosis

Microscopic Examination: Usually IBK is diagnosed by clinical signs. In case of doubt, direct microscopic examination of ocular exudate shows typical Gram-negative organisms. A fluorescent antibody test is also available.

Culture Characteristics: *Moraxella* grows well on blood agar and produces grayish-white colonies surrounded by a narrow zone of beta hemolysis. The organism does not grow on MacConkey agar.

Treatment

The infection can be controlled with antibiotics applied directly to the eye in the form of lotion or ointment. Powders should be avoided because they can further irritate the cornea. Subconjunctival injection of antibiotics and/or corticosteroids also is effective.

Public Health Significance

Moraxella bovis is transmissible to people. Veterinary technicians should wash their hands after handling infected cattle and should consult a physician if their eyes subsequently become red and irritated.

12

Gram-Negative Anaerobic Bacilli

Family: Bacteriodaceae
Genus: *Fusobacterium*
Genus: *Bacteroides*

Among the species of *Fusobacterium*, only one is of veterinary importance.

Fusobacterium necrophorum (*Spherophorus necrophorus*)

General Characteristics

This organism is usually a long, filamentous, Gram-negative bacillus with a beaded appearance. Short rods or coccoid forms also may occur. They are nonspore forming and nonmotile. They prefer anaerobic conditions with 10% CO_2 but may grow in the presence of air.

Mode of Transmission

Direct contact and inhalation of aerosol are the most common modes of transmission for this organism.

Fusobacterium Infections

Calf Diphtheria: The organism invades tissues of the mouth, cheek, gums and tongue to cause brown necrotic tissue covered by a thin membrane. Necrotic epithelium may slough, leaving an ulcer. The disease may spread to cause necrotic laryngitis, characterized by loud wheezing.

Foot Rot of Cattle and Sheep: The affected foot is hot, swollen and painful. The animal is severely lame because of necrotic areas between digits. The organism affects connective tissue and, rarely, horny structures.

Liver Abscesses: The organism invades the rumen wall after inflammation caused by excessive carbohydrates in the feed, then migrates via the portal vein to the liver and produces abscesses.

In horses it causes gangrenous dermatitis of the lower limbs after prolonged exposure to damp, muddy conditions.

Laboratory Diagnosis

Direct microscopic examination of clinical swabs shows the typical organism. The lesions are quite characteristic, with a very foul odor.

Treatment

Treatment involves use of sulfonamides and antibiotics for foot rot; scrubbing the foot and paring away necrotic tissue are very important. Footbaths of iodine and copper sulfate are useful.

Control

A high-roughage diet helps control abscess formation in the liver. Good husbandry is used to control calf diphtheria. Affected animals should be isolated.

Bacteroides nodosus

There are several species of this genus, and most are regarded as opportunistic. However, *Bacteroides nodosus* causes a specific disease in domestic animals.

General Characteristics

These organisms are Gram-negative, slightly curved or straight, nonmotile rods. Methylene blue stain shows red-staining granules at either end of the rod. *Bacteroides nodosus* causes contagious foot rot, a synergistic infection of *B nodosus* and *F necrophorum* in sheep. The disease is characterized by weight loss, lameness, and detachment of a large portion of hoof horn from underlying soft tissues. It is very contagious, and the discharge from the foot is the main source of infection. Disease outbreaks occur more often in spring and autumn during warm weather.

Laboratory Diagnosis

Microscopic Examination: Direct microscopic examination of stained smears shows typical organisms. The fluorescent antibody test is useful.

Treatment

Trimming the foot and swabbing it with formalin are effective. All affected animals must be isolated from healthy ones, and suspected carriers must be sold for slaughter. New additions to the herd should be considered infected, and suspects should be checked by a veterinarian. Lame sheep arriving at auction must be checked for foot rot. It is a reportable disease and, if diagnosed in a flock, results in quarantine and rigorous treatment procedures.

13

Spiral and Curved Bacteria

Campylobacter (Vibrio) Species

General Characteristics

These are Gram-negative, slender, motile, non-spore-forming, slightly curved rods that appear as spiral, comma or seagull shapes in cultures. The organism is microaerophilic or anaerobic, and oxidase positive, indole negative and catalase positive. They do not ferment carbohydrates.

Campylobacter fetus ss *venerealis*

Campylobacter fetus ss *venerealis* causes abortion, irregular heat cycles, and infertility in cattle and sheep. It does not produce pyometra. Bulls show no visible signs of infection, except poor condition from repeated breeding.

Mode of Transmission

This is a true venereal disease that is spread from cow to cow by the bull during breeding and by artificial insemination when contaminated semen and equipment are used.

Laboratory Diagnosis

Microscopic Examination: Direct microscopic examination of aborted fetal tissues or a cotyledon smear reveals typical Gram-negative rods in various forms.

Culture Characteristics: Culture from the aborted fetus stomach contents on blood agar produces grayish-white, nonhemolytic colonies. The organism grows best at 25 C in an N_2 and CO_2 atmosphere. Samples for cotyledons and cervical vaginal mucus are usually contaminated, and isolation of the organism may be difficult.

Serologic Examination: The cervical mucus agglutination test in females and fluorescent antibody tests on preputial washes in males are useful tests. Table 1 summarizes biochemical identification and differentiation.

Treatment

Streptomycin and chlortetracycline are effective. In bulls, flushing with antibiotics is useful.

Control

Effective control procedures include removing infected bulls from the herd, and treating semen with antibiotics before use in artificial insemination.

Campylobacter fetus ss *fetus*

Campylobacter fetus ss *fetus* causes sporadic abortion in cattle, usually in the last trimester of pregnancy.

Mode of Transmission

The organism is transmitted by ingestion and not by coitus.

Laboratory Diagnosis

Laboratory diagnosis of this organism is the same as for *Campylobacter fetus* ss *venerealis*, except this organism can grow in media containing 10% glycine.

Public Health Significance

Campylobacter fetus ss *fetus* may cause abortion and undulant fever-like syndrome in people.

Campylobacter fetus ss *jejuni*

Campylobacter fetus ss *jejuni* is similar to the other 2 members of this genus except for its inability to grow at 25 C. This organism is thermophilic and grows best at 42 C. It causes hemorrhagic mucoid enteritis or winter dysentery in cattle, hemorrhagic enteritis in young dogs, swine dysentery in piglets and enteritis in people.

Laboratory Diagnosis

Culture Characteristics: This organism can be cultured from feces on Balser's Campy-BAP medium containing sheep blood, vincomycin, polymixin B sulfate, trimethoprim lactate, cephalothin and amphotericin B. Incubation in a 10% CO_2 atmosphere produces flat, glossy, spreading colonies along the inoculation streak. Table 1 summarizes biochemical tests used to differentiate *Campylobacter* species.

Public Health Significance

The organism is secreted in milk and feces of cattle. Outbreaks of human disease are usually traced to consumption of contaminated milk.

Table 1. Biochemical tests to differentiate *Campylobacter* species and subspecies.

Species	Host	Catalase	1% Bile	H$_2$S TSI	1% Glycine	3.5% NaCl	Growth at 25 C	42 C	Pigment
C fetus ss *venerealis*	Cattle	+	+	−	−	−	+	−	Tan
ss *intestinalis*	Cattle, sheep	+	+	−	+	−	+	−	Tan
ss *jejuni*	Cattle, sheep	+	+	−	+	−	−	+	Gray-tan
C sputorum ss *sputorum*	People	−	+	+	+	−	+	−	Yellow
ss *bubulus*	Cattle, sheep	−	−	+	+	+	v		Yellow
C mucosalis	Swine	−	−	+	+	+	−	−	Yellow
C fecalis	Cattle, sheep	+	v	+	+	−	v	+	Gray-tan

v = variable reaction

Campylobacter mucosalis
Campylobacter sputorum ss *mucosalis*

Campylobacter mucosalis causes intestinal adenomatosis, hemorrhagic enteritis and necrotic ileitis in pigs.

Laboratory Diagnosis

Table 1 summarizes biochemical tests used to differentiate *Campylobacter* species.

14

Actinomycetes and Related Organisms

Actinomyces Species

General Characteristics

Actinomyces organisms are Gram-positive, filamentous rods that may show branching resembling that of fungi, but mycelia are not formed. Cells may be rod shaped, diphtheroid or coccoid. They are nonspore forming, and most species are anaerobic and catalase negative. The genus *Actinomyces* comprises 3 species, only one of which is of major veterinary importance.

Actinomycosis

Actinomyces bovis causes lumpy jaw in cattle and fistulous withers or poll evil in horses. *Actinomyces suis* and *A bovis* cause granulomatous and suppurative mastitis in sows. *Actinomyces viscosus* causes chronic granulomatous pleuritis with pyothorax and accumulation of pleural and pericardial fluids in dogs.

Actinomyces bovis

Actinomyces bovis causes actinomycosis or lumpy jaw in cattle. This disease is characterized by swelling of the maxilla or jaw, abscesses, granulomas, loose teeth and fistulous tracts.

Mode of Transmission

The organism is naturally found in the mouth and gastrointestinal tract. Infection is initiated by minor wounds or injuries.

Laboratory Diagnosis

Microscopic Examination: Direct examination of pus in a Petri plate reveals "sulfur granules" about 2 mm in diameter. They are larger than the gray-white granules of *Actinobacillus*. For microscopic examination, the granule is crushed on a slide, Gram-stained and examined under oil. *Actinomyces bovis* appears as a club-shaped, long, beaded, filamentous organism.

In liquid media, masses of Gram-negative rods and branching filaments are commonly seen.

Culture Characteristics: This organism grows well anaerobically on blood agar and produces rough modular colonies that are difficult to pick up from the medium. Radiating mycelia can be seen under low power. Table 1 summarizes biochemical tests used for differentiation of *Actinomyces bovis* from other species.

Table 1. Biochemical tests used to differentiate *Actinomyces* species and *Nocardia*.

	Actinomyces bovis	Actinomyces viscous	Nocardia asteroides
Oxygen requirement	anaerobic	aerobic	aerobic
Catalase	–	+	+
Lactose	+	+	–

Treatment

Excision of small, circumscribed lesions is the treatment of choice. In other cases, lesions should be drained and debrided. Prolonged therapy with antibiotics and sulfa drugs is useful.

Dermatophilus congolensis

General Characteristics

These organisms consist of Gram-positive branching hyphal elements. Mycelial filaments commonly fragment to yield coccoid or elongate elements that are usually nonmotile.

Dermatophilus congolensis causes dermatophilosis or strep-tothricosis, characterized by acute or chronic dermatitis involving superficial layers of the skin. In horses and cattle there is matting of the hair, as if painted with a brush, and scab formation. Removal of the scab reveals exudation or moist areas. Areas commonly affected are the back and heels. In sheep, scab formation affects wool quality and causes "lumpy wool." The lower legs may be affected, causing "strawberry foot rot," in which the crusted inflammatory swelling on the feet bleeds readily.

Mode of Transmission

Transmission of this organism is not clearly understood. High ambient temperature, high humidity, a wet environment and ectoparasites may predispose to infection.

Laboratory Diagnosis

A Gram-stained smear of a sample obtained from the moist undersurface of the scab shows typical hyphae.

Treatment

Animals usually recover from the disease without treatment. Chronically affected animals can be successfully treated with penicillin and streptomycin.

Control

Control measures include isolating affected animals, culling infected animals, controlling ectoparasites, and external application of such disinfectants as copper sulfate and cresol.

Nocardia asteroides

General Characteristics

These organisms are Gram-positive, acid-fast, nonspore-forming, nonmotile, aerobic rods with delicate, branching hyphae. The only species of veterinary importance is *Nocardia asteroides*.

Nocardia asteroides causes systemic and local infections in dogs. Systemic infection is characterized by fever, soreness, dyspnea, and enlarged abdomen and lymphadenitis that resembles tuberculosis. The local form is characterized by numerous superficial abscesses that rupture and form fistulas. Similar syndromes are reported in cats. The principal disease in cattle is mastitis. In affected animals, the udder becomes enlarged and firm, and contains blood clots.

Mode of Transmission

The main route of infection is by inhalation or inoculation.

Laboratory Diagnosis

Microscopic Examination: Direct microscopic examination of Gram-stained or acid-fast-stained smears of pus reveal typical Gram-positive branching filaments, or beaded rods. Small whitish granules may be found in pus.

Culture Characteristics: The organism grows well on blood agar and Sabouraud's agar. Growth is best at 25 C or 37 C. The organism requires 4-5 days to grow.

Treatment

Localized lesions should be excised or drained, depending on the lesions. Streptomycin and potentiated sulfa drugs are useful if used for a prolonged period.

Family: Mycobacteriaceae
Genus: *Mycobacterium*

General Characteristics

Mycobacterium organisms are Gram-positive, thin, straight rods that are nonmotile, nonspore forming and aerobic; a 5% CO_2 atmosphere enhances their growth. The organism stains acid-fast positive. It grows slowly and requires 3-4 weeks before colonies are visible. Special medium containing egg yolk is used. Colonies are dry and thickened, and "heap up" to produce a cauliflower-like appearance. The organism grows best at 37 C, except for avian strains.

Pathogenicity

Pathogenicity is related to the organism's high waxy content, which resists phagocytosis. Also, each type of tubercle bacillus contains several proteins that elicit a tuberculin reaction. *Mycobacterium* is rich in lipids that are responsible for most of the cellular tissue reactions and for acid-fastness.

Mycobacterium bovis

Mycobacterium bovis usually causes chronic disease characterized by lesions in the lungs and lymph nodes of the head and thorax of cattle. Lesions are caseocalcareous masses. General signs of the disease are weakness, anorexia, dyspnea and emaciation. Calves fed milk containing bacilli develop lesions in the abdominal cavity rather than the thorax. Chickens are susceptible to the avian type, and most lesions are found in the liver.

Mode of Transmission

Droplet inhalation is the main route of infection in older animals, and ingestion of contaminated feed in younger animals. Stabled animals are more prone to infection due to crowding. Other routes of infection are congenital via the umbilical vein, genital through the penis or female genital tract, and cutaneous through the skin.

Laboratory Diagnosis

Microscopic Examination: Microscopic examination of acid-fast-stained smears reveals acid-fast small rods.

Culture and Other Procedures: Culturing procedures are difficult and not commonly used. Biologic tests are helpful to differentiate *Mycobacterium* strains. Though culture and biologic methods are available to diagnose the disease, most veterinarians use the intradermal tuberculin test.

Treatment

Treatment is not attempted, as it is not economical. Affected animals are usually killed to prevent spread of the disease.

Control

The United States and Canada have eradication programs based on tuberculin testing and slaughter of positive animals.

Public Health Significance

Mycobacterium bovis is transmissible to people. The most common route of infection is ingestion of contaminated milk.

Mycobacterium paratuberculosis

Mycobacterium paratuberculosis causes Johne's disease, characterized by weight loss and chronic diarrhea in cattle, sheep and goats. In dairy cattle there is also a drop in milk production.

Laboratory Diagnosis

Microscopic examination of rectal scrapings or feces shows acid-fast bacilli. Because the organism grows very slowly, culture methods are considered too time consuming. Intradermal tests are of doubtful value.

Treatment

No effective treatment is available.

Corynebacterium Species

General Characteristics

Corynebacterium organisms are small, Gram-positive, pleomorphic rods usually found in arrangements resembling Chinese letters or palisades. They are nonspore forming. Most species are nonmotile and aerobic or microaerophilic. Most are catalase positive and clubbed at one or both ends.

Actinomyces (Corynebacterium) pyogenes

This organism is widespread and is the most important animal pathogen causing pyogenic processes in cattle, sheep, goats and pigs. It is a secondary invader and usually appears only after considerable amount of damage has occurred. Following trauma, abscesses are frequently formed that contain *A pyogenes*. The abscesses contain a greenish to yellowish or white pus with a very foul smell. In older lesions, the abscess develops a thick fibrous capsule that contains an odorless pus.

Other infections caused by this organism include metritis, endocarditis, liver abscesses and mastitis in recently fresh cows. With mastitis the udder is swollen and painful, and contains foul-smelling greenish, yellowish to white pus.

Mode of Transmission

This organism resides in the skin and mucous membranes. The common mode of infection is endogenous. Exogenous infection is through inhalation and direct contact.

Laboratory Diagnosis

Microscopic Examination: Smears of pus reveal small Gram-positive rods arranged as Chinese letters or a palisade pattern.

Culture Characteristics: The organism grows well on blood agar and produces beta hemolysis around pinpoint translucent colonies that are visible after 36-48 hours of incubation. It liquefies gelatin and ferments a number of sugars (Table 2).

Treatment

Treatment of this disease is very disappointing because of inability of antibiotics to penetrate the fibrous tissue capsule. Treatment should be aimed at drainage of the lesion.

Corynebacterium renale

Corynebacterium renale causes pyelonephritis. The incidence of disease is higher in females and occurs near parturition. It develops as an ascending infection from the urethra to the bladder and kidney. Polyuria develops and urine contains white blood cells, blood clots and typical *Corynebacterium* organisms.

Laboratory Diagnosis

Demonstrating organisms in the blood-stained turbid urine is useful. Urea is used for differentiation from other *Corynebacterium* species (Table 2).

Treatment

Penicillin is the drug of choice, but recurrence of disease is quite common.

Corynebacterium pseudotuberculosis

Corynebacterium pseudotuberculosis causes caseous lymph-adenitis in sheep. The disease occurs in dry areas of the western United States, Canada and Australia. The typical lesion is caseous, especially in the superficial lymph nodes.

Laboratory Diagnosis

On blood agar, the colonies are dry and scaly (Table 2).

Treatment

The organism is sensitive to penicillin. In advanced stages, however, treatment is unsuccessful.

Control

Control centers around reducing wounds during shearing, culling old animals, isolating affected animals, and using autogenous vaccines to prevent abscess formation.

Table 2. Biochemical tests used to differentiate *Corynebacterium* species.

Organism	Hemol	Litmus milk	Cata	Urea	Gluc	Mal	Lac	Gel Lique
Actinomyces (*Coryn*) *pyogenes*	Beta	Acid	–	–	+	+	+	+
Coryn renale	–	Alkaline	+	+	+	–	–	–
Coryn pseudo-tuberculosis	Beta (slight)	–	+	+	+	+	+	+
Rhodococcus (*Coryn*) *equi*	–	–	+	v	–	–	–	–
Eubacterium (*Coryn*) *suis*	–	Alkaline	–	+	v	+	–	–
Coryn bovis	–	–	+	+	+	+	–	–

v = variable reaction
Hemol = hemolysis
Cata = catalase
Urea = urease

Gluc = glucose
Mal = maltose
Lac = lactose
Gel Lique = gelatin liquefaction

Rhodococcus (Corynebacterium) equi

Rhodococcus equi causes infectious pneumonia in foals. The disease occurs in summer and late spring. Ulcers occasionally develop in the intestinal wall. There are lesions in the cervical lymph nodes, as with strangles.

Laboratory Diagnosis

Direct microscopic examination of Gram-stained smears from clinical specimens or colonies shows coccoid organisms containing metachromatic granules. The organism is encapsulated, catalase positive and nonhemolytic, and has no action on litmus milk (Table 2).

Treatment

Sulfonamides and penicillin are useful.

Control

Hygienic measures and isolation of infected animals aid control of infection.

Corynebacterium bovis

Corynebacterium bovis is a minor cause of mastitis.

Eubacterium (Corynebacterium) suis

Eubacterium suis is the only anaerobic organism in this genus. It causes cystitis and pyelonephritis, and is thought to be transmitted during coitus.

15

Cell Wall-Free Bacteria

Mycoplasma Species

General Characteristics

Mycoplasma organisms are Gram negative, pleomorphic, nonflagellated, oxidase negative and catalase negative, and use arginine as their source of energy. They are resistant to penicillin because they have no cell wall. Mycoplasmas are the smallest free-living cells between viruses and bacteria. They grow on synthetic media; however, they need a complex medium containing serum and yeast cells. Colonies on complex agar medium are minute and tend to grow into the agar, giving them a "fried-egg" appearance.

Mode of Transmission

Infection by *Mycoplasma* species may be endogenous or exogenous. Generally, exogenous infections are transmitted by inhalation of contaminated droplets.

Mycoplasma Infections

Mycoplasma infections are generally characterized by a slow spread and chronic nature, with epithelial or serosal surfaces affected. Antibiotics fail to eliminate the infection.

M mycoides: This organism causes contagious pleuropneumonia in cattle, characterized by a fever and pleuropneumonia.

M agalactiae: This mycoplasma causes contagious agalactia and arthritis in sheep and cattle. Clinical signs include total agalactia of the affected gland and nonsuppurative arthritis with painful swelling of affected joints.

M bovis: This organism causes severe mastitis.

M bovigenitalium: This mycoplasma has been associated with mastitis and genital tract infections.

M dispar: It causes pneumonia in cattle.

M synoviae: This organism causes synovitis in birds.

M hyopneumoniae: It causes enzootic pneumonia in pigs. The infection persists for many months or even years.

M hyorhinis: This organism has been isolated from nasal cavities and pneumonic lungs of swine.

M hyosynoviae: This mycoplasma causes arthritis in older pigs.

Ureaplasma Species

Ureaplasma hydrolyses urea, distinguishing it from *Mycoplasma*. *Ureaplasma urealyticum* causes calf pneumonia, vaginitis and abortion in cattle.

Laboratory Diagnosis

Mycoplasma and *Ureaplasma* are identified by colony characteristics and inhibition of the growth of the colonies by specific antisera (impregnated discs).

Fluorescent antibody techniques, metabolic inhibition tests and other biochemical tests are used for specific identification.

16

Aerobic and Anaerobic Spirochetes

Family: Leptospiraceae
Leptospira Species

General Characteristics

Leptospira organisms are unflagellated, tightly coiled spiral rods with a rotating corkscrew type of motility. The organism is difficult to stain, but is considered Gram-negative. The organism is an obligate aerobe. The optimal pH for growth is 7.4, and optimal temperature is 28-30 C. Dark-field or phase-contrast microscopy is used to demonstrate these bacteria in clinical fluids. The organism has an affinity for silver stains, and special silver staining procedures are used to observe the organism in tissues. *Leptospira* organisms are the smallest of the spirochetes.

Mode of Transmission

Urine from infected animals is the principal source of infection. The disease is usually acquired through broken skin and mucous membranes and, to a lesser degree, by ingestion of contaminated feed.

Leptospiral Infections

Cattle: Leptospira pomona and *L hardjo* cause localized renal infection in cattle. In young animals, the disease is characterized by fever, anorexia, dyspnea and hemoglobinuria. In older cattle, no hemoglobinuria develops and the disease goes undetected until the animal aborts. Abortion usually occurs in the latter part of pregnancy. There is also decreased milk production.

Swine: Leptospira pomona, L canicola and *L icterohemorrhagiae* cause subclinical or asymptomatic disease.

Dog: Leptospira canicola causes fever, depression, anorexia and jaundice. Frequent urination and nephritis are also seen.

Laboratory Diagnosis

Microscopic Examination: Dark-field, phase-contrast or fluorescent-antibody microscopic examination of urine reveals *Leptospira* organisms.

Serologic Examination: These organisms grow very slowly and require special growth media, so serologic diagnostic methods are commonly used. Paired acute and convalescent serum samples should be examined to determine antibody titers. Fluorescent antibody techniques are useful. The agglutination lysis test may be useful. Mixing killed *Leptospira* (antigen) and serum containing specific antibodies results in a clumping reaction.

Animal Inoculation: Intraperitoneal inoculation of guinea pigs and hamsters, followed by inoculation of blood tissues from these animals into culture medium, improves the chances of isolating organisms.

Treatment

Streptomycin, penicillin and tetracycline are very effective if given early in the disease.

Control

Susceptible animals should be vaccinated with a *Leptospira* bacterin. The bacterin is often included in multivalent vaccines. Animals shedding the organisms should be culled. Replacement stock should be carefully screened.

Public Health Significance

It is contracted by people by drinking raw milk, contact with infected animals, and swimming in contaminated water.

Family: Spirochaetaceae
Treponema hyodysenteriae

General Characteristics

Treponema are flagellated, tightly coiled, obligate anaerobic, oxidase-negative organisms that stain poorly with Gram stain.

Mode of Transmission

Ingestion is the main route of infection.

Treponema Infections

Treponema hyodysenteriae causes dysentery in feeder pigs. The disease is characterized by bloody diarrhea, fever and anorexia. The animal may die as a result of dehydration and toxemia.

Laboratory Diagnosis

Gram staining a direct smear of intestinal material shows typical organisms.

Treatment

Gentamicin, lincomycin and nitromidazole appear to be most effective. No vaccine is available.

Borrelia Species

General Characteristics

Borrelia is a loosely coiled, flagellated, microaerophilic organism that stains poorly (negative) with Gram stain.

Mode of Transmission

Borrelia is transmitted by the bites of ticks or through droppings containing the microorganisms.

Borreliosis

Borrelia anserina causes borreliosis in birds in many tropical countries in the world. The disease is characterized by fever, yellow-greenish diarrhea, drowsiness and emaciation.

Laboratory Diagnosis

Dark-field microscopic examination of wet blood smears demonstrates actively motile spirochetes.

Treatment

Penicillin and tetracycline are effective.

Control

A bacterin made from chicken embryo is widely used.

Borrelia burgdorferi

Borrelia burgdorferi causes borreliosis or Lyme disease in dogs. Transmission is through the bite of various *Ixodes* ticks. The disease is characterized by fever, inappetence, lethargy, lymphadenopathy and acute onset of lameness or pain. A chronic form of the disease is characterized by recurrent, intermittent, nonerosive arthritis.

Laboratory Diagnosis

Attempts to culture *B burgdorferi* is the laboratory are usually unsuccessful. Use of monoclonal antibodies for positive identification is necessary. Both indirect fluorescent antibody assay and enzyme-linked immunosorbent assay (ELISA) are used to diagnose Lyme disease.

Treatment

Tetracycline and ampicillin are used to treat acute cases. Chronic cases are more difficult to treat.

Control

Control is centered around rapid removal of ticks from dogs. No vaccine is available.

Public Health Significance

Though there is no evidence to show that Lyme disease is transmissible from dogs to people, people can become infected by the bite of the same tick that infects dogs.

17

Obligate Intracellular Bacteria

Family: Rickettsiaceae
Rickettsia rickettsii

General Characteristics

Rickettsia are Gram-negative, small, pleomorphic, nonflagellated rods or cocci. They are usually found intracellular (within host cells) but may be facultatively extracellular.

Rickettsia rickettsii causes Rocky Mountain spotted fever in people, rodents, rabbits and horses. Horses are the main reservoir of the organism. The organism is transmitted to people by ticks that feed on infected animals. In dogs, *R rickettsii* causes tick fever, signs of which include fever, depression, anorexia and hyperesthesia. Lymphadenitis and edema of the legs and dependent skin may also develop.

Laboratory Diagnosis

An indirect fluorescent antibody test should be interpreted in light of clinical signs.

Coxiella burnetti

Coxiella burnetti causes Q fever in people and mastitis in cows. The disease is usually acquired from its reservoirs in infected cows, sheep, goats and rodents by direct contact. This organism is the most heat resistant of all pathogenic bacteria and forms the basis for temperature requirements for pasteurization of milk.

Family: Chlamydiaceae
Chlamydia psittaci

General Characteristics

Chlamydia psittaci organisms are tiny, obligate intracellular elementary bodies. They cause psitticosis in birds, characterized by nasal discharge, dullness, sleepiness or depression. They also cause enzootic abortion in ewes, polyarthritis in cows, and diarrhea in calves that do not receive colostrum.

Laboratory Diagnosis

Chlamydiosis is diagnosed by isolation of the organism in chicken embryos or cell culture, and with the complement fixation test. A 1:16 titer is considered positive.

Control

All birds entering the United States and Canada must be quarantined for 30-45 days and fed chlortetracycline in the feed.

References

Chapters 6-17

1. Blood DC *et al*: *Veterinary Medicine*. 6th ed. Bailliere Tindall, London, 1983.

2. Buchanan RE *et al*: *Bergey's Manual of Determinative Bacteriology*. 8th ed. Williams & Wilkins, Baltimore, 1974.

3. Carter GR: *Essentials of Veterinary Bacteriology and Mycology*. 3rd ed. Lea & Febiger, Philadelphia, 1986.

4. Fraser CM *et al*: *The Merck Veterinary Manual*. 8th ed. Merck, Rahway, NJ, 1986.

5. Timoney JF *et al*: *Hagan and Bruner's Microbiology and Infectious Diseases of Domestic Animals*. 8th ed. Cornell Univ Press, Ithaca, NY, 1988.

6. Kreeg NR and Holt JF: *Bergey's Manual of Systematic Bacteriology*. Williams & Wilkins, Baltimore, 1984.

7. Carter GR and Chengappa MM: Keeping up with the changes in bacterial and fungal nomenclature. *Vet Med* 84:256-260, 1989.

18

Classification of Fungi

Classification of Fungi

Fungi are classified by microbiologists or biologists for convenience of reference and communication. As with any classification system, fungal classification is subject to constant revision. A simplified form of fungal classification is presented in Figure 1.

Phylum: Zygomycota

Fungi in this phylum have aseptate (coenocytic) mycelia (Fig 2). Asexual reproduction is by production of sporangiospores, and sexual reproduction by the fusion of 2 compatible hyphae and formation of a zygospore. Many members of this phylum are animal pathogens, such as *Rhizopus*, a cause of reproductive problems.

Phylum: Ascomycota

Fungi in this phylum have septate mycelia (Fig 2). Sexual reproduction is by ascospores (sexual spores) produced in a sac-like structure called an ascus. Asexual reproduction occurs through a variety of asexual spores, predominantly conidia (*eg*, *Aspergillus*), or by budding or fission, as seen in many yeasts (*eg*, *Saccharomyces cerevisae*).

Phylum: Basidiomycota

Fungi in this phylum have septate mycelia (Fig 2). These are the most complex fungi and include mushrooms, rusts and smuts. They reproduce by sexual spores called basidiospores on the surface of specialized structures called basidia. Very few members of this phylum are animal pathogens.

Phylum: Deuteromycota (Fungi Imperfecti)

Fungi in this phylum have septate mycelia and thallospores (chlamydospores, arthrospores, blastospores) (Fig 2). They reproduce asexually by producing conidia. They are not known to reproduce by sexual processes. This group includes many economically and medically important fungi.

Figure 1. A simplified system of classification of fungi.

Aseptate Mycella	Septate Mycella
Phylum: Zygomycota	Phylum: Ascomycota
• Includes saprophytic molds	• Includes molds and yeasts
• Sexual spores – zygospores	• Sexual reproduction by ascospores
• Asexual spores – sporangiospores	
	Phylum: Basidiomycota
	• Sexual reproduction by basidiospores. Mainly plant pathogens.
	Phylum: Deuteromycota
	• Includes molds, yeasts and dimorphic fungi
	• Asexual reproduction only
	• Conidia and various types of vegetative spores produced
	• No sexual spores

Figure 2. Structural and reproductive characteristics of 4 phyla of fungi.

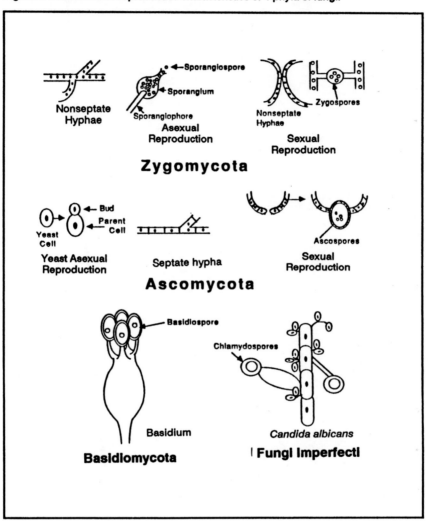

19

Structure and Physiology of Molds

Molds are multicellular fungi. They form tubular filaments called hyphae, and contain no chlorophyll. The hyphae may be septate. A tangled mass of hyphae is called a mycelium. Molds produce cottony growth on organic matter.

Structure of Molds

Molds have a rigid cell wall of chitin, which is primarily cellulose in composition. The nucleus is surrounded by a membrane. Mitochondria have oxidative activity.

Physiology of Molds

All molds are strictly aerobic. Molds require less moisture than bacteria. When the environment gets very dry, fungi (including molds) produce spores.

Molds can grow in a wide range of pH, from 2 to 9. The optimal pH for most species is 5-6. Their temperature requirement varies greatly, ranging from 0 to 60 C. The optimal range for most species is 22-30 C.

All molds are Gram positive. A special stain called lactophenol cotton blue (LPCB) is commonly used for staining molds. Their growth curve is similar to that of bacteria (Chapter 3, Fig 8).

Mold spores are not as heat resistant as bacterial spores, and can be very easily destroyed by heat. Some molds produce inhib-

itory compounds that inhibit the growth of other organisms. For
example, *Penicillium* produces penicillin that inhibits growth of
many Gram-positive bacteria.

Reproduction of Molds

Fungi (molds) can reproduce by asexual and sexual methods
(except fungi imperfecti). Generally, asexual reproduction is
more important for propagation of the species and may be
categorized as follows:

Fragmentation of somatic cells, with each fragment growing
into a new individual.

Fission of somatic cells.

Budding of somatic cells, with each bud producing a new
individual.

Production of spores, with each spore usually germinating to
form a germ tube that develops into a mycelium.

The most common form of asexual reproduction in molds is
by formation of various types of spores (Fig 1).

Conidiospores

These are formed at the free end of hyphae and arise in the
form of long chains at the tip of sterigma. There are 2 types of
conidia:

Microconidia: These are conidiospores of various shapes.
They arise directly from hyphae (Fig 1). An example of a fungus
reproducing by conidiospores is *Aspergillus*.

Macroconidia: These are large, multicompartmented cells of
various shapes (Fig 1). They originate from the conidiospore as
singles, pairs or clusters.

Sporangiospores

Sporangiospores are produced in a specialized, sac-like structure called a sporangium (Fig 1). Sporangia are produced from
the terminal portion of a stalk or special hypha called a sporan-
giophore. When the sporangium breaks, the spores are set free.
Mucor is an example of a fungus reproducing by sporangio-

Figure 1. Common types of fungal spores.

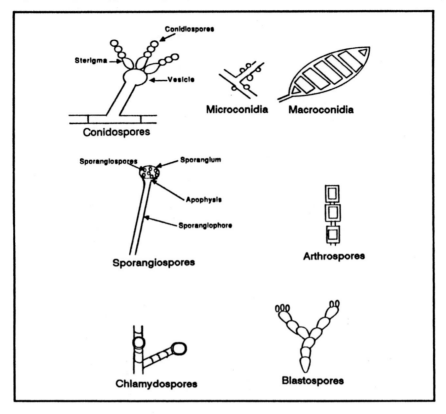

spores. These spores can also be produced by sexual reproduction.

Arthrospores

These spores are produced by constriction and fragmentation of hyphae, resulting in rectangular spores with thickened cell walls (Fig 1).

Chlamydospores

Chlamydospores are thick-walled spores formed by rounding off and enlargement of certain hyphae (Fig 1). Some members of Ascomycota produce these spores.

Blastospores

These spores are produced by budding from the tip of a mycelium, either as single spores or as small clusters of spores (Fig 1).

20

Structure and Physiology of Yeasts

Yeasts are unicellular, spheroid, oval or rod-shaped fungi. They do not form hyphae and contain no chlorophyll.

Structure of Yeasts

The capsule of yeasts is composed of slimy material that surrounds the cell wall composed chiefly of chitin or yeast cellulose. The nucleus is eucaryotic. Mitochondria show oxidative activity. Yeasts contain granules for storage of energy.

Physiology of Yeasts

Yeasts can be aerobic or anaerobic. They require vitamin B to initiate growth. After growth has begun, the yeast can produce its own vitamin B.

Yeasts require more moisture than bacteria for growth. They can grow in a pH ranging from 3 to 9.5. The optimal pH is between 4.5 and 5. Most require a minimum temperature of 22-25 C for growth. Pathogenic species require 37 C.

All yeasts are Gram positive. Their growth curve is similar to that of bacteria (Chapter 3, Fig 8).

Reproduction of Yeasts

Yeast reproduce by asexual or sexual means. Asexual reproduction is by budding or fission.

Figure 1. Asexual reproduction of yeasts.

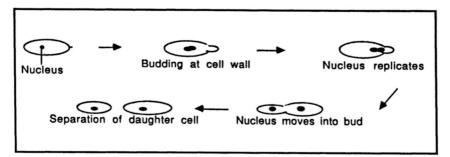

Figure 2. Sexual reproduction of yeasts.

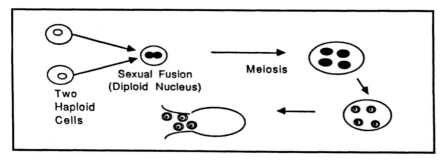

Budding is the most common method of asexual reproduction in yeast. In budding, a portion of the cell wall bulges out to form the bud. The nucleus in the mother cell divides and one of the daughter nuclei moves into the bud. When the bud is fully formed, the bud separates from the mother cell (Fig 1). At times, clumps or chains of cells may be seen.

In reproduction by fission, the cell divides by transverse binary fission, as in bacteria.

In sexual reproduction, sexual union of 2 yeast cells forms a diploid nucleus (Fig 2). This undergoes meiosis to form 4 daughter nuclei. Each of these nuclei forms a thick wall around itself and becomes a spore. The original cell cytoplasm disappears and its cell wall becomes a sac or ascus containing 4 spores. When the ascus ruptures, the spores are released, and each spore grows into one new yeast cell in a suitable environment.

References

Chapters 18-20

1. Carter GR: *Essentials of Veterinary Bacteriology and Mycology*. 3rd ed. Lea & Febiger, Philadelphia, 1986.

2. Delaat ANC: *Microbiology for the Allied Health Professions*. Lea & Febiger, Philadelphia, 1973.

3. Pelczar MJ *et al* : *Microbiology*. 4th ed. McGraw-Hill, New York, 1977.

4. Ross FC: *Introductory Microbiology*. 2nd ed. Merrill Publishing, Columbus, OH, 1986.

5. Rebell G and Taplin D: *Dermatophytes*. 4th ed. Univ Miami Press, Coral Gables, FL, 1979.

6. Whittaker RH: New concepts of the kingdom of organisms. *Science* 163:150-160, 1969.

21

Fungi and Disease

Fungi are saprophytes, and their pathogenicity is accidental and much more diverse than that of bacteria and viruses. They cause disease in 3 ways. They can directly invade healthy tissues of a host to cause systemic and subcutaneous mycoses. They can also produce toxic substances that, when ingested, cause disease, as in mycotoxicosis. Finally, they can produce sensitizing substances, such as allergens or spores, to cause disease.

Endogenous infections involve species of fungi that are commensals in the animal's body and cause disease when the host's defense system is compromised, as from debilitating disease or long-term use of corticosteroids.

Exogenous infections are caused directly or indirectly by contact with infected animals, fomites or lesions. To cause disease, the fungus must come in contact with and enter the host. The portals of entry in most cases are by deposition of fungal spores or infective material directly or indirectly onto the host, inhalation of fungal spores, or ingestion of fungal spores.

Host Defenses and Fungal Infection

The skin offers an effective barrier to infection, but minor trauma or injuries facilitate invasion. The digestive tract is fairly resistant to primary invasion by fungi, though many spores may survive passage through the digestive tract. Inhalation depends on the size of the spores. Only very small spores reach the lower respiratory tract when inhaled.

22

Laboratory Procedures in Mycology

Direct Microscopic Examination

For direct microscopic examination of clinical specimens, the specimen is mixed with a few drops of 10% KOH on a glass slide and a coverslip is applied. The slide is placed on top of a moistened paper towel in a Petri dish and the dish is covered to keep the specimen from drying out. It is allowed to sit overnight for complete digestion of background debris, hair and scales by the KOH. This clears the background and makes it easier to observe fungal elements. The slide is then examined for spores, hyphae or other fungal elements characteristic of fungi (see Chapter 18).

Molds are generally filamentous. The filaments are called hyphae, and a mass of hyphae is called the mycelium. Yeasts are not filamentous. Molds and yeasts are generally much larger than bacteria. Each fungus has characteristic fungal elements that can be compared to illustrations and descriptions in a reference book for identification.[2,5,6]

Staining the sample may also help identify the fungus. Gram, Giemsa, Wright or lactophenol cotton blue stains are used. Acid-fast, periodic acid-Schiff and silver-methenamine stains may also be used if specific fungi are suspected.

Sample Collection

Cleaning the skin site before collection of samples for dermatophyte culture may remove the best sample material, so the area should be cleaned as little as possible. Lightly wiping or soaking with 70% alcohol reduces bacterial and saprophytic fungal contamination but does not entirely eliminate dermatophytes. Iodine should not be used, as it may completely destroy any dermatophytes.

To select the sample, choose broken hairs or pieces of the underside of a crust. Also, scrape the surface of a lesion that is lightly scaled over or take scrapings of affected nails. The sample should be obtained from the periphery of the lesion, that is, the growing edge, rather than from the center of the lesion.

Types of clinical specimens that may be submitted for examination are skin scrapings (hair, scales), mucosal surface scrapings, tissue samples, purulent exudate from infected tissues, granulomatous lesions, and body fluids, such as milk and cerebrospinal fluid.

Culture

Both molds and yeasts grow well on agar too acidic for good growth of bacteria. Sabouraud's agar is a commonly used culture medium for fungi. It may be poured on plates, or into tubes or bottles. Use of tubes or bottles is best because the number of spores released when the container is opened is fewer than with use of plates. Fungi grow more slowly than do bacteria and the plates, if used, should be taped shut to prevent desiccation (drying). Increased moisture in the incubation environment is also provided with some culture techniques. It is common to incubate fungal cultures at room temperature, but some species are grown at 37 C. The cultures are allowed to incubate for 21-30 days.

Sabouraud's C&C agar is also widely used instead of, or in addition to, plain Sabouraud's agar. It contains chloramphenicol, an antibiotic that inhibits bacterial growth on the medium, and cycloheximide, which inhibits contaminant fungal growth.

Potato flake agar can be used instead of Sabouraud's. It is inexpensive and easy to make, using instant potato flakes and agar. Chloramphenicol and cycloheximide are added to this.

When growth appears, usually in 5-8 days, the gross colonial appearance (morphologic characteristics and pigmentation) is noted. Final identification is by microscopic examination of the spores and mycelia or other fungal elements. The aerial growth is removed by sterile technique and placed in a few drops of lactophenol cotton blue stain, and a coverslip is applied for microscopic examination.

Fungassay Dermatophyte Test Medium: Fungassay Dermatophyte Test Medium (Pitman-Moore) is supplied in individual bottles. Use of this medium helps confirm the diagnosis of dermatophyte infections (ringworms). Pathogenic fungi, such as *Microsporum canis, Microsporum gypseum* and *Trichophyton mentagrophytes*, cause a color change in the medium from amber to red, usually within 72 hours and in less than 10 days. Growth of dermatophytes produces alkaline products that cause the color of the acidic medium to change.

The medium contains inhibitors that suppress growth of most bacteria, yeasts and contaminant fungi, but the same color change may occasionally be produced by a heavy contamination of saprophytic fungi or bacteria. Dermatophytes cause the color change with (or before) their colony growth. In contrast, saprophytic fungi grow into visible, well-established colonies before the color changes, usually after 10 days. In addition, dermatophyte colonies are usually light colored and saprophyte colonies are usually dark colored. Bacteria can be differentiated from fungi by their morphologic appearance. Microscopic examination of the fungal growth can be done for further identification.

Wood's Lamp Examination

Use of ultraviolet rays from a Wood's lamp may help identify a dermatophyte infection. Some dermatophytes fluoresce under the ultraviolet light. A positive reaction is a bright yellow-green fluorescence of broken hairs or scales. Plucked hairs are examined for fluorescence at the follicular end of the hair. False-positive fluorescence may be caused by *Pseudomonas* species, scales, lint, sebum, dandruff, crusts and topical medications. The absence of fluorescence does not rule out dermatophytosis, as it may be caused by a fungus that does not produce fluorescent metabolites.

It is most useful to use the Wood's lamp to choose particular hairs for microscopic examination and culture.

23

Fungi Causing
Superficial Mycoses

Dermatophytes are a group of closely related filamentous fungi that invade dead tissues of the skin. Dermatophytes are erosive in nature and do not penetrate deeper than the skin. The lesions are typically circular; hence the term "ringworm" is used to describe dermatophyte infections. Two important genera of veterinary importance are *Microsporum* and *Trichophyton*.

Superficial Mycoses
(Dermatophyte Infections)

Microsporum canis is the principal dermatophyte affecting dogs and cats. Young animals are most often affected. The infection is acute and lesions are scattered. The usual site is the head, particularly the ears and eyes. The trunk and limbs may also be affected. Lesions consist of discrete, circular areas of hair loss, with scaling and heavy crusting. Other species causing ringworm infection in dogs and cats are *Trichophyton mentagrophytes* and *M gypseum*.

Trichophyton verrucosum is the main dermatophyte affecting cattle. *Trichophyton mentagrophytes* and other species may cause ringworm in cattle. Lesions are usually found on the head and neck but may be scattered across the body, legs and tail. Coin-sized or larger crusted lesions resemble a patch of asbestos. Removal of the crust reveals a moist, bleeding area.

The most common dermatophyte affecting horses is *Trichophyton equinum*. Dry, scaly circular lesions and loss of hair give the animal a "moth-eaten" appearance. Lesions are common in the saddle area.

Microsporum nanum causes ringworm in pigs. The hair is not usually affected, but skin scales contain hyphae.

Trichophyton mentagrophytes and *T verrucosum* affect sheep. Lesions are confined to the head and neck.

Mode of Transmission

The main reservoir of dermatophytes is infective debris shed from the animal. Infection is usually through deposition of infectious skin debris on skin that has suffered a minor injury.

Laboratory Diagnosis

In large animals, skin scrapings are obtained from the periphery of the lesion with a blunt scalpel. The hair should be plucked, never cut. In small animals, the animal is examined with Wood's lamp in a completely dark room. Affected hair may fluoresce a bright yellow-green color. Hairs are plucked for culture and microscopic examination. If no fluorescing hairs are seen, scrape or pluck hairs from the periphery of the lesions and examine or culture. Keep in mind that only 40% of *Microsporum canis* specimens fluoresce; therefore, negative results with a Wood's lamp does not eliminate the possibility of infection. Microscopic examination of hair and skin scrapings is done by placing a specimen on a glass slide and adding a drop of 10% NaOH.

Location of Spores

Ectothrix: Ectothrix spores are located outside the hair shaft, as in *M gypseum* and *M nanum*, or arranged in a regular chain, as in *T mentagrophytes*, *T equinum* and *T verrucosum*.

Endothrix: Endothrix spores are confined within the hair shaft, as in *T mentagrophytes*, which has both ectothrix and endothrix spores.

Culture

Sabouraud's agar is not satisfactory for isolation of dermatophytes from heavily contaminated material. Mycobiotic medium is Sabouraud's medium to which antibiotics have been added for inhibition of growth of contaminating bacteria and saprophytic fungi.

Dermatophyte test medium (Fungassay: Pitman-Moore) is commercially available and suitable for a clinic laboratory. The test medium contains phenol red as an indicator. The amber color of the medium changes to red with dermatophyte growth. It is not satisfactory for *T verrucosum* as it does not contain thiamin, inositol or yeast extract, which are absolute growth requirements for this dermatophyte. Direct microscopic mounts of fungal growth reveal characteristic dermatophyte structures.

Treatment

Griseofulvin is the drug of choice but is too expensive for large animal use, and has a number of side effects.

Public Health Significance

Microsporum canis, *M nanum* and most species of *Trichophyton* are transmissible to people.

Microsporum Species

General Characteristics

Macroconidia occur frequently and are spiny (Fig 1). Spores are of the ectothrix type.

Microsporum canis

Microsporum canis is one of the most important dermatophytes and accounts for 90% of all feline and 70% of canine ringworm cases.

Microscopic Morphology

Large numbers of macroconidia are seen. They are large, spindle shaped, frequently rough, and thick walled, with a knob at one end (Fig 1). Macroconidia contain more than 6 compartments or cells. Microconidia are few and are usually sessile on the hyphae.

Colony Morphology

Colonies appear as a white, coarsely fluffy thallus that usually develops a characteristic deep yellow pigment on the underside, referred to as "reverse pigment."

Diagnostic Features

Characteristic macroconidia and yellow-orange reverse pigment are produced.

Microsporum gypseum

Microscopic Morphology

Numerous macroconidia are present. They are large, ellipsoid structures with a thin-walled, rough surface and usually containing less than 6 compartments (Fig 1). The macroconidia are shorter and broader than those of *Microsporum canis*.

Colony Morphology

Colonies appear as a rapidly spreading thallus with a coarse powdery surface and a cinnamon-brown color in the center. Reverse pigment is usually dull yellow, tan to yellow-cream colored.

Diagnostic Features

Characteristic macroconidia and colony morphology are produced.

Microsporum nanum

Microscopic Morphology

Macroconidia are rough walled and egg shaped to ellipsoid, consisting of only 1-3 cells (Fig 1).

Colony Morphology

Colonies appear as a spreading thallus with a powdery dark buff surface. The reverse pigment is reddish brown.

Figure 1. Morphologic characteristics of common dermatophytes.

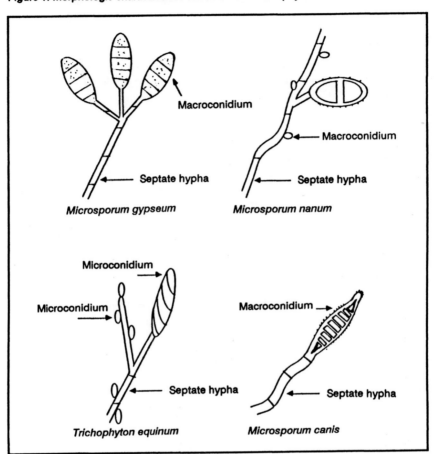

Diagnostic Features

Macroconidia and reverse pigment are diagnostic.

Trichophyton Species

General Characteristics

Macroconidia are seen less commonly, thin walled and not spiny. The location of spores is ectothrix and endothrix.

Trichophyton mentagrophytes

Microscopic Morphology

Macroconidia are scarce. They are cigar shaped and multi-celled, with thin smooth walls. Small spherical microconidia resembling clusters of grapes grow in bunches along the length of hyphae (Fig 2). Tightly wound spirals may be numerous.

Colony Morphology

Trichophyton mentagrophytes produces a flat thallus with a cream to white cottony powdery surface that has the appearance of face powder sprinkled in concentric rings and rays. The reverse pigment is dark red, yellow to rose.

Diagnostic Features

Colony morphology and small round conidia and coiled spirals are diagnostic.

Figure 2. Morphologic characteristics of *Trichophyton* dermatophytes.

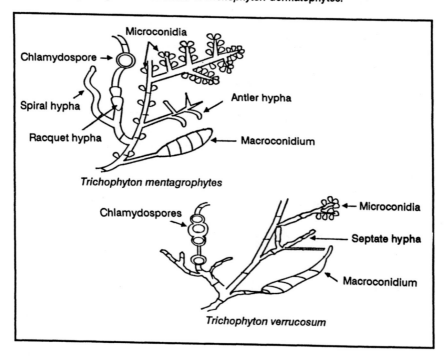

Trichophyton equinum

Microscopic Morphology

Macroconidia are very rare. They have thin smooth walls and less than 6 compartments (Fig 1). Microconidia are thin and elongated.

Colony Morphology

The colony is flat but develops folds with age. The surface is at first white, and later becomes velvety cream to tan. Reverse pigment varies from bright yellow to deep red-brown.

Diagnostic Features

Colony morphology, reverse pigment and elongated microconidia are diagnostic.

Trichophyton verrucosum

Microscopic Morphology

On Sabouraud's agar, tortuous hyphae with chlamydospores are seen. On thiamin-enriched medium, the mycelium is more regular and has numerous microconidia. Macroconidia are extremely rare and 3-5 celled, with thin smooth walls (Fig 2).

Colony Morphology

Colonies usually appear as a white slow-growing thallus, heaped up and button-like. On enriched medium, the thallus is spreading, flat and downy.

Diagnostic Features

These include the morphology of the thallus and absolute requirements for thiamin, inositol or yeast extract. Cultures are slow growing. Growth is improved at 37 C.

24

Fungi Causing Deep Mycoses

In this group are included all mycotic infections that involve subcutaneous and systemic mycoses.

Fungi Causing Subcutaneous Mycoses

Sporothrix schenckii

General Characteristics

Sporothrix is a dimorphic fungus. At 25 C it is mycelial, consisting of a septate mycelium with sessile conidia. At 37 C it is a budding yeast.

Sporothrix schenckii causes sporotrichosis, which is a chronic infection characterized by subcutaneous nodules involving the lymphatics. The nodules eventually ulcerate to the surface and discharge pus. The lymph nodes are also enlarged. This disease is more commonly seen in horses.

Laboratory Diagnosis

Microscopic Examination: Microscopic examination of pus and tissue is not usually helpful. Cigar-shaped and pleomorphic yeast cells can be best observed by the fluorescent antibody technique.

Culture Characteristics: Plating pus onto Sabouraud's agar and incubating at room temperature for a week produces wrinkled white to black colonies.

Animal Inoculation: Diagnosis can be confirmed by intraperitoneal inoculation of mice and demonstration of cigar-shaped or pleomorphic yeast in the peritoneal exudate.

Systemic Mycoses

Histoplasma capsulatum

General Characteristics

Histoplasma is a dimorphic fungus. At 25 C it produces mycelia consisting of septate hyphae with small pear-shaped microconidia. Under adverse conditions and on old cultures, it produces large, spherical clock-faced macroconidia. At 37 C it is a budding yeast.

Histoplasma capsulatum causes histoplasmosis, the most common systemic mycosis of dogs. It affects the reticuloendotholial system, and causes coughing, weight loss, diarrhea and an enlarged liver.

Laboratory Diagnosis

Microscopic Examination: Examination of a peripheral blood buffy coat smear stained with Wright's stain shows oval yeast cells in monocytes.

Culture Characteristics: Culture on Sabouraud's agar at 37 C produces membranous white colonies. At room temperature they form cottony mycelia with characteristic macroconidia.

Public Health Significance

Histoplasma capsulatum is transmissible to people through saliva, vomitus, feces and urine.

Pathogenic Yeasts

Cryptococcus neoformans

General Characteristics

Cryptococcus is a spherical or ovoid, thick-walled budding yeast. At 25 C it is a yeast, and at 37 C it develops a capsule that can be stained with India ink.

Cryptococcus neoformans causes cryptococcosis, a subacute or chronic disease of dogs, cats, cattle, sheep, goats, horses and people. The organism causes mastitis in cattle, respiratory disease in dogs and cats, and localized paranasal granulomas in horses. It does not respond to antibiotic treatment.

Mode of Transmission

Cryptococcus neoformans occurs widely in nature, especially in pigeon droppings. Most cases of cryptococcosis result from inhalation or ingestion of yeasts.

Laboratory Diagnosis

Microscopic Examination: Wet mounts of purulent nasal discharge show budding yeasts but no capsule. If stained with India ink, the capsule can be seen (Fig 1).

Culture Characteristics: On Sabouraud's agar, whitish or cream-colored colonies are produced. Other cryptococci do not grow at 37 C.

Treatment

Amphotericin B and ketoconazole are effective.

Public Health Significance

Cryptococcus neoformans is transmissible to people.

Candida albicans

General Characteristics

Candida is an oval budding yeast that produces a thick-walled chlamydospore when grown on cornmeal agar.

Candida albicans causes candidiasis. Animals are predisposed to infection by poor nutrition, use of corticosteroids, physiologic changes, extensive use of antibiotics, and immunologic disorders. In poultry, it is a major problem in young birds. Affected birds are listless and have reduced feed intake due to lesions in the mouth and esophagus. In other animals, gastrointestinal and mucocutaneous involvement produces pseudomembranous lesions. In people it causes oral and vaginal thrush.

Figure 1. *Cryptococcus neoformans.*   Figure 2. *Candida albicans.*

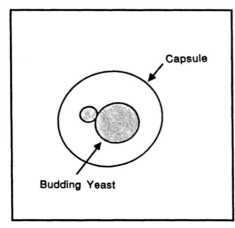
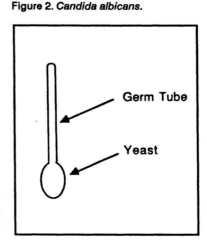

Laboratory Diagnosis

Microscopic Examination: Direct microscopic exam of wet mounts or Gram-stained specimens reveals a budding yeast-like morphology or chains of blastospores producing pseudomycelia.

Culture Characteristics: On blood or Sabouraud's agar, *Candida albicans* produces cream-colored pasty and smooth colonies with a yeast-like odor. In the germ tube test, *C albicans* inoculated into human or bovine serum and incubated at 37 C for 2-4 hours produces small sprouts called germ tubes developing from yeast cells (Fig 2). On chlamydospore or cornmeal agar, *C albicans* produces characteristic filamentous growth, with thick-walled chlamydospores that are essential for its identification. To confirm the diagnosis, send samples to reference laboratories for carbohydrate assimilation and histopathologic examination.

Treatment

Antimycotic drugs, such as ketoconazole, are effective for topical application. Nystatin in the feed and water is effective in prevention or treatment of candidiasis in chickens.

Public Health Significance

Candida albicans is transmissible to people by inhalation, and causes respiratory and CNS signs.

Blastomyces dermatitidis

General Characteristics

Blastomyces is a dimorphic fungus growing in mycelial form at 25 C and a broad-based budding yeast at 37 C.

Blastomyces dermatitidis causes blastomycosis, which is most common in the north-central and southeastern United States. In dogs, the lung is the primary organ affected; granulomatous lesions give it a mottled appearance. Clinical signs include weight loss and ocular and nasal discharge. Respiratory signs vary from coughing to dyspnea. The disease is transmitted through inhalation of spores.

Laboratory Diagnosis

Microscopic Examination: Wet mount examination of clinical specimens from discharging ulcers or granulomatous lesions in 20% KOH-treated smears reveals the characteristic thick-walled yeast form of the organism.

Culture Characteristics: Cultured on Sabouraud's agar and blood agar at 25 C shows septate hyphae, with typical oval or pyriform conidia. Thick-walled budding yeasts are similar to those observed by direct smears and are seen at 37 C.

Animal Inoculation: Intraperitoneal inoculation of hamsters or mice with a heavy saline suspension of yeast or mycelial forms yields typical yeast cells in peritoneal fluid after 21 days.

Coccidioides immitis

General Characteristics

Coccidioides is characterized by nonbudding thick-walled spherules or sporangia containing granular material or small endospores. When cultured on solid medium, the mycelial phase produces thick-walled, rectangular or barrel-shaped arthrospores. Usually the mycelial phase does not occur in tissues.

Coccidioides immitis causes coccidioidomycosis, which is primarily a respiratory disease. The lungs are the main organ involved and clinical signs include a harsh dry cough, fever and weight loss. Ocular signs may also be present. Coccidioidomyco-sis is a dust-borne noncontagious disease. Infections are most prevalent in desert areas of the southwestern United States, Mexico, and Central and South America.

Laboratory Diagnosis

Microscopic Examination: Direct microscopic examination of a KOH wet mount reveals typical spherules in tissue. For fluo-rescent antibody staining of tissue, send samples to reference laboratories.

Culture Characteristics: Cultures on Sabouraud's agar at 25 C produce barrel-shaped arthrospores that are highly infec-tious. *Do not* attempt cultures of *Coccidioides* unless you have experience working with this organism.

Public Health Significance

Infected animals are not considered public health hazards. However, handling mycelial cultures is dangerous.

25

Opportunistic Filamentous Fungi

There are 4 filamentous fungi of veterinary importance. They are referred to as monomorphic because they exhibit only a fungal form. The sporangia of *Mucor* arise directly from mycelia. The sporangia of *Rhizopus* arise from nodes on horizontal hyphae (stolons). The sporangia of *Absidia* arise from internodes on stolons.

Lesions produced by *Mucor, Rhizopus* and *Absidia* are granulomatous and ulcerative. In cattle, lesions occur in the abomasum and in the aborted fetus. In pigs, lesions are gastric ulcers and granulomas. Nasal granulomas are seen in horses.

Aspergillus fumigatus is one of the most common fungal species affecting animals. In cattle, abortion follows infection of the lungs. Upper respiratory disease is seen in horses. In dogs, the nasal form localizes in the sinuses. Brooder pneumonia occurs in chicks and pullets.

Laboratory Diagnosis

Microscopic Examination: Direct examination of granulomatous tissue in KOH wet mounts reveals septate hyphae.

Culture Characteristics: *Aspergillus fumigatus* is a rapidly growing fungus. As the thallus grows and the conidia develop, the thallus becomes bluish-green and powdery. Cellophane tape is used to examine the fruiting head and differentiate it from *Penicillium* spp, which have a broom-type fruiting head.

Serologic Examination: Serologic tests on nasal swabs are useful.

Histopathologic Examination: Histopathologic examination of tissue or lesions preserved in 10% formalin reveals septate hyphae invading tissues.

Treatment

Treatment involves surgical curettage of lesions, and use of amphotericin B and other antimycotic drugs.

Public Health Significance

Aspergillus fumigatus causes lung infections in people.

26

Fungi Causing Mycotoxicoses

Mycotoxicosis is an intoxication caused by ingestion of food contaminated by toxins produced by fungi. Some toxin-producing fungi are *Aspergillus, Fusarium, Claviceps* and *Penicillium*.

The main source of mycotoxins in animals is stored grains. Factors influencing production of toxins in stored grains are high humidity, high ambient temperatures, and contamination with field mold. Damaged grains are most susceptible to mold invasion.

Clinical Signs

The degree of toxicity varies with the dose of toxin ingested, and age and species of animal involved. In most cases the disease is not recognized clinically and is manifestd as poor growth. Salivation, depression, anorexia, kidney and liver damage, increased blood clotting time, and reproductive problems are some nonspecific signs.

Control

Control centers around not feeding moldy hay, destroying moldy feed, or diluting moldy feed with normal feed (3:1). Feed should be stored properly to prevent moldiness.

CHAPTER 26

References

Chapters 21-26

1. Blood DC *et al*: *Veterinary Medicine*. 6th ed. Bailliere Tindall, London, 1983.

2. Carter GR: *Diagnostic Procedures in Veterinary Bacteriology and Mycology*. 4th ed. Charles C Thomas, Springfield, IL, 1979.

3. Fraser CM *et al*: *The Merck Veterinary Manual*. 8th ed. Merck, Rahway, NJ, 1986.

4. Timoney JF *et al*: *Hagan and Bruner's Microbiology and Infectious Diseases of Domestic Animals*. 8th ed. Cornell Univ Press, Ithaca, NY, 1988.

5. Jungerman PF and Schwartzman RM: *Veterinary Medical Mycology*. Lea & Febiger, Philadelphia, 1972.

6. Rebell G and Taplin D: *Dermatophytes*. 4th ed. Univ Miami Press, Coral Gables, FL, 1979.

27

Classification of Viruses

A virus is an obligate intracellular parasite because it requires a living cell to multiply. As with many other microorganisms, viruses have been identified as agents of disease. Rabies, cowpox, influenza and AIDS are some of the diseases caused by viruses. What are viruses? How do they differ from bacteria? What is their classification system?

Classification of Viruses

Viruses are classified by their hosts as bacterial (bacteriophage), plant or animal viruses. They can also be classified by their physical and chemical properties. Nuclear material may be composed of DNA or RNA, but not both. This system of classification will be used for discussing viral infections in this text.

Size and shape are also constant for particular groups of viruses. The presence or absence of an envelope (capsule) can also be used in classification.

28

Morphology and Replication of Viruses

Structure of Viruses

Viruses are composed of an inner core of nucleic acid, a protein coat, and an outer capsule (Fig 1).

Nucleic Acid

Nucleic acid may be RNA or DNA (Fig 1). This is the infectious part of the virus that stores genetic information. It is used for making protein found in the viral coat, for making enzymes required to invade the host, for replicating the viral nucleic acid, and for directing the host cell to make viral parts and assemble them into complete virus particles.

Protein Coat

The protein coat is called the capsid, and consists of protein subunits called capsomers (Fig 1). It protects the nucleic acid core from enzymatic digestion and other destructive factors in the environment, aids infection by interacting with host receptor sites to promote attachment to susceptible host cells, and confers specificity to the virus. It is antigenic in nature.

Capsule

The capsule is a membranous envelope that surrounds the protein coat and is composed of lipids or lipoprotein. Some enveloped viruses have virus-specific glycoprotein spikes (Fig 1). The capsule aids attachment of the virus to susceptible host cells, helps it escape normal body defense mechanisms by making it look like a host cell, and protects the nucleic acid core.

Viruses may be helical, icosahedral, enveloped or complex (Fig 1).

Figure 1. The structure of viruses.

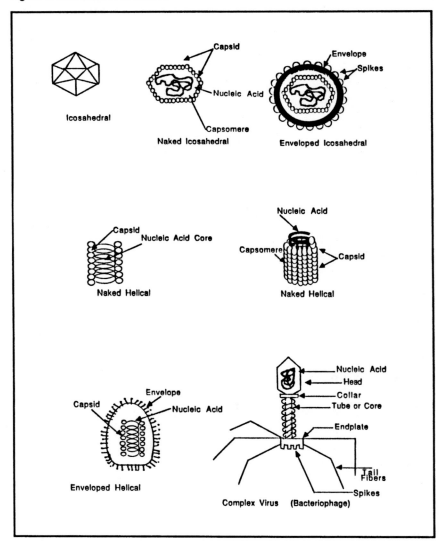

Helical viruses resemble a long rod. They have a capsid, which is a hollow cylinder surrounding the nucleic acid core.

An *icosahedral virus* resembles a polyhedron, with 20 triangular facets or sides (Fig 1).

Enveloped viruses have a capsid or protein coat surrounded by a membranous envelope. An enveloped helical virus is rabies virus. An enveloped icosahedral virus is infectious bovine rhinotracheitis virus.

Complex viruses are a combination of helical and polyhedral forms, with leg-like or plate-like structures. An example is a bacteriophage (Fig 1).

Viruses can pass through micropore filters that do not allow passage of bacteria. They range in size from 20 μ to 300 μ.

Replication of Viruses

Animal Viruses

Animal viruses replicate in a complex series of steps (Fig 2):

Attachment: Before a virus can enter a cell, it must attach or adsorb itself to the specific receptor sites on the host cell. This process is very cell specific.

Figure 2. Replication of an enveloped DNA virus.

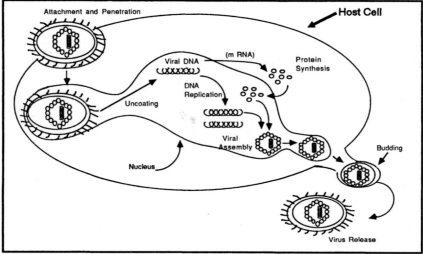

Penetration: The entire virus enters the cell by a process called viropexis or endocytosis.

Uncoating: This refers to release of viral nucleic acid into the host cell. After uncoating, viral DNA enters the cell nucleus, where it is replicated. In the case of RNA viruses, nucleic acid needs only to enter the cytoplasm of the cell to be replicated. Since the process of uncoating is very complex and varies from virus to virus, it will not be discussed in detail in this text.

Latent Period (Eclipse): This is a noninfective period that ranges from 3 to 15 hours, depending on the type of viral nucleic acid.

Replication: Viral nucleic acid directs the host cell to manufacture viral nucleic acid, protein, enzymes and other viral parts.

Virus Assembly: Newly produced nucleic acid and protein are assembled into the new mature virus. Viral parts that are not assembled remain in the host cell as inclusion bodies, for example, the cellular inclusion bodies (Negri bodies) seen in rabies.

Virus Release: The new virus particle is released from the cell by lysis of the cell or budding from the cell wall.

Bacterial Viruses

A bacteriophage is a bacterial virus. The bacteriophage consists of a hexagonal head containing nucleic acid, a rigid tail, a contractile sheath, and a tail fiber (Fig 1).

The steps involved in bacteriophage replication are similar to those for animal viruses (Fig 3). The entire bacteriophage does not enter into the bacterium. Rather, the bacteriophage, using its tail structure like a syringe, injects DNA into the bacterium. After viral DNA is in the host cell, the virus directs the host's metabolic machinery to manufacture specific viral particles. The viral parts are then assembled into a complete virus, which is released from the cell to infect other host cells.

Differences Between Viruses and Bacteria

There are many differences between viruses and bacteria:

- Bacteria grow in artificial media, but viruses do not. Viruses require living cells to reproduce.

Figure 3. Replication of a bacteriophage.

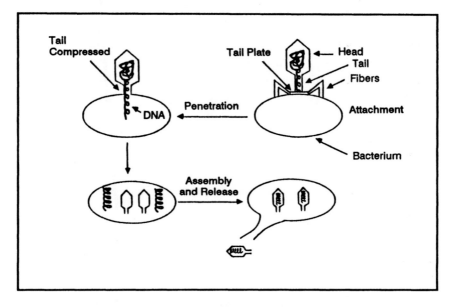

- Bacteria have cellular organelles and metabolize, but viruses do not.
- Bacteria increase in size and divide by binary fission; viruses do not. Viruses cannot replicate or reproduce on their own. After entry into a living host cell, the virus directs the cell's metabolic machinery to replicate viral DNA and make other viral parts and assemble them into a finished virus.
- Bacteria contain both DNA and RNA, whereas viruses have only DNA or RNA but never both.
- Viruses do not contain ribosomes.
- Viruses do not respond to antibiotics, which are effective against bacteria.
- Viruses are sensitive to interferons (a protein synthesized by virus-infected host cells that stops viral replication), while bacteria are not.

Interferon

Interferon inhibits viral multiplication. It does not block entry of the virus into the cell. Rather, it acts on uninfected cells so that they produce antiviral protein that stops viral replication without affecting cellular function.

Types of Interferon

Alpha: This type of interferon is produced by virus-infected leukocytes. It is species specific, that is, if it is produced in dog cells, it will only protect dogs against a variety of viral infections.

Beta: This type of interferon is produced by virus-infected fibroblasts. It is also species specific.

Gamma: This type of interferon is derived from antigen-stimulated T-cells. It has broader applications, is not host cell specific, and can offer protection between species.

Properties of Interferons

Interferons are not virus specific and can be used against a variety of viral infections. They are composed of protein or glycoprotein, and are stable in acids and, therefore, can be administered by oral routes.

They are heat stable, weak antigens, nontoxic to cells, produced in very small quantities and are difficult to purify, which makes their clinical use very limited.

References
Chapters 27-28

1. Atlas RM: *Basic and Practical Microbiology*. Macmillan, New York, NY, 1986.

2. Cano RJ and Colome JS: *Microbiology*. West Publishing, St. Paul, MN, 1986.

3. Fenner F *et al*: *Veterinary Virology*. Academic Press, Orlando, FL, 1987.

4. Roberts WA and Carter GR: *Essentials of Veterinary Virology*. Michigan State Univ Press, East Lansing, 1981.

29

Laboratory Procedures in Virology

Diagnostic virology has become an important segment of modern veterinary medicine. Though it is unlikely that you will perform diagnostic virology procedures, aside from collecting specimens, a brief overview of some virology procedures is given for your information.

Specimen Collection

Containers: Sterile swabs, vials containing virus transport medium, bottles for feces or other samples that do not require transport medium, blood collection equipment for both serum and plasma samples, and bottles containing fixative for histologic examination are the most typical containers used for collection of virus samples.

Timing: Collect the specimen for viral analysis as soon as possible after the onset of clinical signs. For serologic tests, 2 blood samples are obtained, one during the acute phase, usually when the animal is seen and clinical signs are obvious, and the second during the convalescent phase, usually 2 weeks after the first specimen is taken. An increased antibody titer may be observed in the second sample.

Collection Site: The collection site depends upon the clinical signs and knowledge of the suspected virus, such as nasal swabs for respiratory diseases, feces for gastroenteritis, or vaginal mucus for abortion.

Transport: Ice or cold packs are used if the ambient temperature is moderate and transit time is less than one day. If temperatures are high or transit time is extended, dry ice may be used.

Special Precautions: If exotic or zoonotic viruses are suspected, special packaging and appropriate permits are necessary for interstate and international transport. This information is available from the postal service, shipping companies, and state veterinary and public health authorities.

Cell Culture

To demonstrate the presence of a virus in a specimen, the virus is grown (isolated) in the laboratory or the viral antigens or antibodies are assayed.

Unlike bacteria, which can be grown on nutrient agar, viruses need living cells in which to grow and replicate. This process of growing viruses on cells is called tissue culture or cell culture.

There are different types of cells from which to choose for tissue culture of viruses. Most animal cells can be grown *in vitro* for at least a few generations, but some cells divide indefinitely and are used for virus isolation. These cells are called continuous cell lines and are of a single type of cell. Continuous cell lines, such as those from fetal kidney, embryonic trachea, skin or other cells, are derived from monkeys, dogs, cattle, pigs, cats, mice, hamsters, rabbits and other animals. The sample is commonly inoculated into a primary culture of cells derived from the same species of animal as the specimen was taken.

After the cell culture has been inoculated with the specimen and incubated, the cell culture is examined. If the virus is present, cell damage may be visible as the viruses "take over" the cells. This damage is referred to as a cytopathic effect. Different types of cytopathic effects are used in identifying viruses. Some viruses cause cell lysis, while others cause the cells to fuse and form syncytia or giant cells. An inclusion body is another type of cytopathic effect that may be seen.

Serologic Examination

Clinical signs and cell culture examination may identify the virus to a family level and perhaps to the genus and species level as well, but definitive identification requires serologic procedures based on immunologic principles. Sometimes these serologic procedures may be used on the specimens directly, which saves the time and expense of cell culture.

Direct Immunofluorescence

In this type of test, an antibody to a specific virus, such as rabies virus, is labeled with a fluorescent dye and added to the specimen. If viral antigen is present in the specimen, the antibody binds to it (Fig 1). If the viral antigen is not present, the antibody is washed away in the rinsing step of the procedure. Upon microscopic examination, any antibody-antigen complex is visible as fluorescence.

Indirect Immunofluorescence

An indirect procedure using 2 antibodies is also used. Antiviral antibodies called immunoglobulins, are produced in an animal, such as a rabbit. The second antibody is an antirabbit immunoglobulin labeled with the fluorescent dye. The second antibody binds to the first antibody, which binds to any viral antigen in the specimen (Fig 2). This complex is then detected on microscopic examination.

If no viral antigen is present in the specimen, there is no binding and the unbound dye is washed away. The technique

Figure 1. With direct immunofluorescence, antiviral antibody labeled with a fluorescent dye is added to the specimen, forming an antibody-antigen-dye complex.

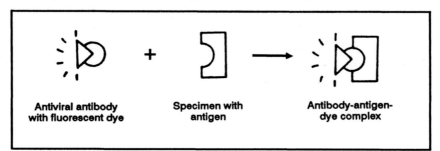

| Antiviral antibody with fluorescent dye | Specimen with antigen | Antibody-antigen-dye complex |

Figure 2. With indirect immunofluorescence, antibody forms a complex with the viral antigen, which then binds with antirabbit immunoglobin and the fluorescent dye.

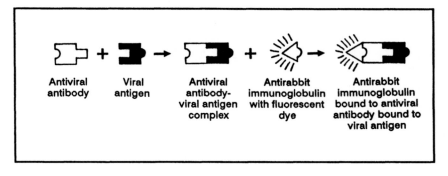

has some advantages over the direct fluorescent technique, such as increased sensitivity. An example of a disease diagnosed by this method is cryptosporidiosis.

Radioimmunoassay

In this procedure, the label is a radioactive element, such as iodine. This radioactive label is attached to an antiviral antibody that combines with viral antigen in the specimen (Fig 3). A gamma counter is needed to detect the presence of the antibody-antigen complexes. Thyroid hormone levels are measured by this method.

Enzyme-Linked-Immunosorbent-Assay

This type of test uses test trays containing antibody-coated wells. The sample is added to the wells and any viral antigen

Figure 3. In radioimmunoassay, antiviral antibody labeled with a radioactive element, such as iodine, is added to the specimen, forming an antibody-iodine-antigen complex.

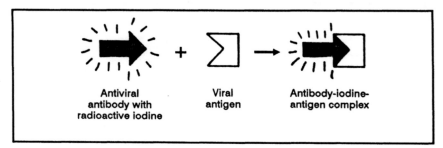

binds to the antibody. A second antiviral antibody is then added; this antibody is enzyme-labeled. If virus was present in the sample and was bound to the antibody that coated the well, the second antibody also binds to the virus. When a substrate that reacts with the enzyme is added, the resultant color change is proportional the amount of viral antigen present in the sample (Fig 4). If there was no virus in the sample, the second antibody is washed away in the rinsing process and no color change is seen. Feline leukemia virus is detected with this method.

Immunodiffusion

With immunodiffusion, antigen in the specimen and antibody are placed into separate wells in agar. They diffuse into the agar and form a visible band of precipitation when they combine (Fig 5). If no band forms, there is no viral antigen present in the sample. Bovine leukemia virus is detected by immunodiffusion.

Complement Fixation

Complement is a series of enzymes in normal serum that combine with an antibody-antigen complex to cause lysis of cells, destruction of bacteria, and other immune responses. In complement fixation, complement becomes "fixed" when it combines

Figure 4. With enzyme-linked immunosorbent assay, viral antigens bind with antibody in the test wells, an enzyme-labeled antiviral antibody is added, and finally a substrate is added to produce a color change.

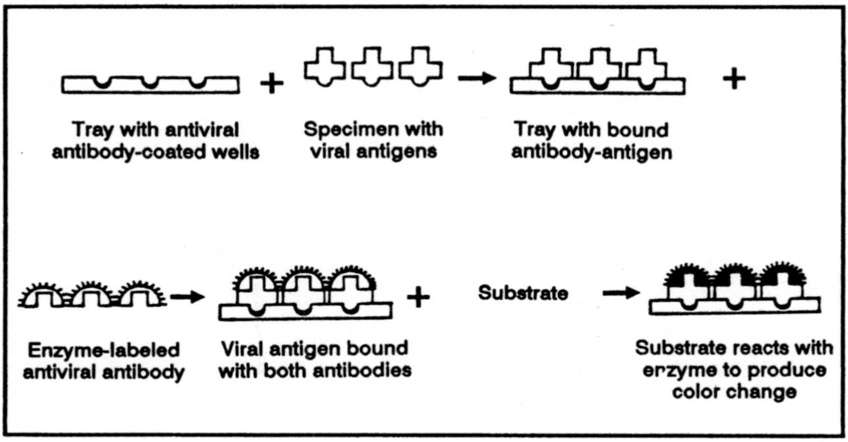

Figure 5. In immunodiffusion, antigen and antibody in separate wells diffuse out into the agar and form a visible precipitate where they meet.

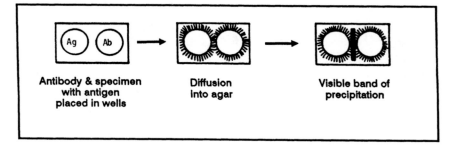

Antibody & specimen   Diffusion   Visible band of
with antigen   into agar   precipitation
placed in wells

with an antibody-antigen complex. The complement fixation test is used to detect viral antibodies in a serum sample, as in anaplasmosis.

The patient's serum sample is heated to inactivate its complement. A known amount of complement is added to the serum. A known amount of viral antigen is then added and this mixture is incubated to allow fixation of the complement if viral antibodies are present in the serum. Sensitized RBCs (RBCs that have complexed with anti-RBC antibodies) are then added and the mixture is incubated. If viral antibody is present in the serum, viral antibody-viral antigen complexes are formed and there is no lysis of the RBCs. Complement was "fixed" and was not available to lyse RBCs. If no viral antibody is present in the serum, complexes of anti-RBC-antibody-RBC-antigen and complement are formed, and the RBCs are lysed (Fig 6).

Virus Neutralization in Cell Culture

Two types of virus neutralization techniques are used: inhibition of cytopathic effects and plaque reduction. Before doing this test, it must be known that the virus in the sample causes cytopathic effects or plaque formation. By using a specific antibody, the virus can then be identified. Bovine virus diarrhea is diagnosed by this method.

Inhibition of Cytopathic Effects: A specific antibody to a particular virus is incubated with a specimen that contains the unidentified virus. Cell culture tubes are then inoculated with

Figure 6. The complement fixation test shows no RBC lysis if viral antibody is present.

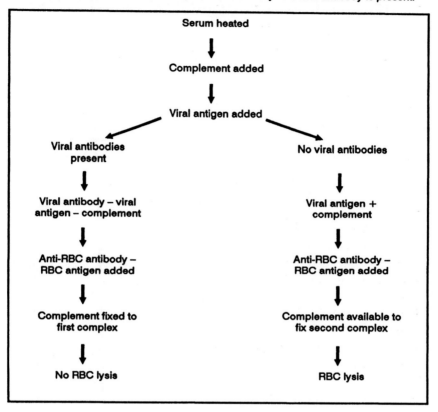

this mixture and checked daily for cytopathic effects. Complete inhibition of cytopathic effects is considered a positive virus neutralizaton test and indicates the identity of the virus. The virus in the specimen formed a complex with the added antibody and was unable to cause cytopathic effects. If cytopathic effects are produced, the particular virus tested is ruled out.

Plaque Reduction: The specimen containing the unidentified virus is incubated with antibody for a particular virus. Cell culture tubes are then inoculated with this mixture and incubated again. An agar medium containing a dye is added and incubated, and the culture is observed daily for the presence and numbers of plaques, which are necrotic cells surrounded by living cells. The necrotic cells do not pick up the dye and are colorless, while living cells are stained by the dye. An 80% or greater reduction of plaque counts is positive and confirms the identity of the virus. The specific antibody has formed a complex with the virus, preventing it from forming plaques.

Electron Microscopy

The 2 basic techniques for routine diagnostic use of electron microscopy are negative staining of virus particles and thin-sectioning of virus-infected cells. Electron microscopy can be used to identify viruses to the family level and sometimes to the genus or species level. Parvovirus can be detected by electron microscopy.

Negative Staining: A virus suspension made from a clinical sample is mixed with a heavy metal stain. The heavy metal atoms surround the virus particles. The electron beam of the electron microscope passes through the virus particles but cannot pass through the metal atoms. This gives the appearance of a "negative stain," that is, the virus is light and "unstained" and the surrounding background of metallic atoms is dark and appears "stained."

Thin-Sectioning: This technique uses the intact virus-infected cells, which are examined with the electron microscope. It gives a more reliable diagnosis than simple negative staining of the clinical sample because tissues from the animal or inoculated tissue cell culture are used, and the viurs and the cell it is infecting are both preserved for examination. This complex procedure consists of several preparatory steps and includes the negative staining step.

Immunoelectron Microscopy

With this technique, monoclonal or polyclonal antibodies are added to a viral suspension made from the clinical specimen. If the corresponding viral antigens are present in the suspension, antibody-antigen complexes form. The suspension is centrifuged and combined with a heavy metal stain and then applied to an electron microscope grid for examination using the negative staining procedure.

Antibody is added to increase the chance of seeing viral particles. The complexes or aggregates are more easily seen than a few individual viruses, especially when viral concentration is low. Coronavirus may be detected by this method.

Direct Detection of Viral Nucleic Acid

In this research technique, DNA strands of a virus are separated and one of the strands is labeled with a radioactive isotope or another nonradioactive label. The labeled "probes" are added to separated strands of viral DNA from cells infected with the unknown virus. Under appropriate conditions, the 2 strands combine with each other if they are from the same virus. Because one of the strands is labeled, it can be detected and the identity of the virus is confirmed.

30

Viruses and Disease

Though it is unlikely that veterinary technicians will use any diagnostic virology techniques in their work, it is important to have some knowledge of viral diseases and their laboratory diagnosis to effectively communicate with the veterinarian and clients. Following is a brief description of common viurses and their role in diseases of veterinary importance.

DNA VIRUSES

Adenoviruses

Adenoviruses are double-stranded DNA, icosahedral, naked viruses that replicate in the nucleus of the host cell.

Infectious Canine Hepatitis

Infectious canine hepatitis (ICH) is an acute viral disease. It is caused by adenovirus type I, which is shed in urine, feces and saliva, and is transmitted by ingestion of infected materials.

Clinical Signs: ICH is more severe in young dogs. In the acute form, clinical signs include fever, vomiting, diarrhea and severe abdominal pain. The animal has pinpoint hemorrhages on the mucous membranes that tend to bleed easily. About a quarter of the dogs that recover develop corneal opacity or "blue eyes." Affected dogs recover or die within 2 weeks.

Treatment and Control: Treatment includes blood transfusions, intravenous fluids, and antibiotics to control secondary infections. Vaccination is effective in preventing ICH. The vaccine is usually incorporated into multivalent vaccines.

Tracheobronchitis

This highly contagious disease of dogs, caused by adenovirus type II, is also called "kennel cough." Other etiologic agents, such as parainfluenza virus or herpesvirus and *Bordetella bronchiseptica*, may also be involved. The disease is more prevalent where large numbers of dogs are kept together, as in boarding and breeding kennels and veterinary hospitals.

Clinical Signs: The history is vital in diagnosis. Dogs recently boarded or in contact with a dog that had the disease are most susceptible. Affected dogs have a harsh, dry, nonproductive cough that is often followed by gagging. People often think that something is "stuck in the dog's throat." Palpation of the trachea produces a cough.

Treatment and Control: Antibiotics are helpful in controlling secondary bacterial infection. Vaccination is effective in controlling kennel cough.

Papillomaviruses

These are double-stranded DNA, icosahedral, nonenveloped viruses. They replicate in the host cell nucleus. The virus is transmitted through open skin lesions.

Warts

Clinical Signs: The virus affects the surface epithelium, causing wart-like lesions. They are more commonly seen in cattle. The incidence is highest in calves and yearlings. Warts can occur on the teat, udder, head, neck and shoulder. In horses they occur around the lips and nose. Sarcoids are similar to warts and occur in horses as skin tumors but do not metastasize.

Treatment and Control: Warts usually regress spontaneously. Autogenous vaccine often helps speed regression.

Parvoviruses

Parvoviruses are single-stranded DNA, icosahedral, naked viruses. They replicate in the host cell nucleus.

Parvoviral Enteritis

Canine parvovirus causes parvoviral enteritis in dogs. Ingestion is the main mode of transmission.

Clinical Signs: Parvoviral enteritis was first recognized in the early 1980s and quickly became widespread. The disease is characterized by vomiting, diarrhea, depression and dehydration. It may progress to hemorrhagic diarrhea and death. In puppies under 8 weeks of age it causes sudden death from myocarditis.

Diagnosis: Fecal samples may be submitted to reference laboratories for hemagglutination testing, virus isolation, enzyme-linked immunosorbent assay (ELISA) and electron microscopy.

Treatment and Control: Treatment is usually supportive and includes fluid therapy and corticosteroids to prevent shock. Control depends on good management. Kenneled dogs should not be overcrowded. Good nutrition and sanitation must be provided. Sick dogs should be isolated. Healthy dogs should be routinely vaccinated.

Feline Panleukopenia

Feline panleukopenia virus causes a highly contagious disease that affects all members of the cat family.

Clinical Signs: The disease is characterized by fever, anorexia, vomiting and dehydration. Diarrhea develops in the later stages. Profound leukopenia leads to secondary bacterial infection. Ocular and nasal discharges may be seen. Recovery or death occurs within a week of onset.

Laboratory Diagnosis: A white blood cell count of less than 3000 WBC/μl is diagnostic of the disease if the animal also has the other clinical signs. For confirmation, submit samples to reference laboratories for virus isolation, fluorescent antibody testing or enzyme-linked immunosorbent assay.

Treatment: Treatment is supportive and includes fluid therapy, antibiotics to combat secondary infection, and good nursing care.

Control: This virus is so widespread that almost all cats are exposed at some time during their lives. Older cats are probably immune. Vaccination is very effective.

Infected cats should be isolated. New cats should be held in isolation for several weeks before introduction into the cattery.

SMEDI

SMEDI is an important viral disease of pigs characterized by reproductive failures including stillbirths, mummification, embryonic death and infertility. Pigs may be born alive and die within a week of birth.

Control: Sows immune to one serotype of SMEDI virus do not provide immunity to others in their colostrum. Control is difficult because the mode of transmission is not clearly understood.

Herpesviruses

These are double-stranded DNA, icosahedral, enveloped viruses. They replicate in the host cell nucleus. The diseases caused by herpesviruses are:

Pseudorabies

Pseudorabies (Aujeszky's disease or "mad itch") is an infectious disease transmitted by ingestion of contaminated material or via minor wounds.

Clinical Signs: In cattle and sheep, the disease is characterized by intense pruritus leading to intense licking and rubbing against objects, resulting in lacerations.

In swine it causes inapparent infection. Pregnant sows may abort. In piglets it causes acute paralysis and death in 24 hours.

Diagnosis: Clinical signs are often diagnostic in cattle. For confirmation, isolation of the virus on tissue culture, animal inoculation, fluorescent antibody staining of frozen tissues, and ELISA are diagnostic tests available.

Control: The disease is controlled by isolating infected cattle, eliminating ingestion of contaminated feed, not commingling cattle with swine, and removing dead carcasses immediately.

Infectious Bovine Rhinotracheitis

This herpesvirus causes an acute contagious disease of the upper respiratory tract of cattle. The mode of transmission is by direct contact for the respiratory form, and contaminated semen for the genital form.

Clinical Signs: The disease is characterized by difficult respiration, excessive salivation, ulcers on the mucous membranes of the nose and esophagus, and bloody diarrhea. Older animals are generally constipated. Abortion may occur. The genital form consists of pustular vulvovaginitis, characterized by pustules.

Diagnosis: IBR infection is diagnosed by clinical signs, virus isolation from nasal swabs, and serologic examination.

Control: IBR can be prevented with the various killed and modified-live vaccines available.

Feline Rhinotracheitis

This virus causes a respiratory disease of cats characterized by fever, sneezing, coughing, mucopurulent nasal discharge and conjunctivitis.

Diagnosis: Diagnosis is by virus isolation from pharyngeal swabs or fluorescent antibody testing.

Treatment: Treatment consists of supportive therapy with tube feeding and IV fluids, and antibiotics to control secondary bacterial infection.

Marek's Disease

This is a progressive disease of chickens in which clinical signs vary. The neurolymphomatosis form is characterized by asymmetric paralysis of one or both legs or wings. Acute Marek's disease is characterized by depression and ataxia, with significant mortality. In the ocular lymphomatosis form, the iris of one or both eyes is gray ("gray-eye" blindness). With cutaneous Marek's disease, there are round, nodular lesions in feather follicles.

Diagnosis: Marek's disease is diagnosed by clinical signs, isolation of virus on tissue culture, and serologic examination.

Control: Vaccination prevents tumor formation but not infection.

Equine Rhinopneumonitis

This is a mild upper respiratory disease of horses that causes abortion. In foals it causes acute respiratory infection.

Clinical Signs: The disease is commonly spread when horses are congregated from different sources, such as shows and sales.

In the respiratory form, clinical signs are more common in young animals. An outbreak of the disease in foals is often followed by abortion in mares. Clinical signs include fever, conjunctivitis, coughing and a runny nose. Abortion occurs 2-4 months after infection.

Treatment: Therapy consists of good nursing care and use of antibiotics to control secondary infection.

Control: Rhinopneumonitis can be controlled by good hygiene, isolation of infected animals, and vaccination.

Avian Infectious Laryngotracheitis

This is an acute, highly contagious disease affecting chickens of all ages, particularly those 4-18 months of age.

Clinical Signs: After an incubation period of 2-8 days, a mild cough, sneezing, ocular discharge, and dyspnea develop. In acute cases, the neck is raised during inspiration, with head shaking and expectoration of bloody mucus.

Diagnosis: Diagnosis is based on clinical signs and postmortem findings characteristic of the disease. It is confirmed by fluorescent antibody staining of smears and tissues, isolation of virus from the chorioallantoic membrane, and observation of intracellular inclusion bodies in tracheal epithelium.

Treatment and Control: Affected animals should be kept quiet. Dust should be controlled and a mild expectorant given as needed. Vaccines should be administered in epizootic areas.

Poxviruses

Poxviruses are the largest and most complex of all viruses. They have double-stranded DNA, are brick shaped and envel-

oped, and replicate in cytoplasm. The important diseases caused
by poxviruses are:

Cowpox

This is a rare eruptive disease of dairy cows that usually
affects the udder and teats. The virus spreads by contact during
milking. Within a few days, vesicles develop into pustules that
may rupture, leaving raw ulcerated areas that scab over.

Diagnosis: Electron microscopic examination of samples
shows the large distinct virus.

Control: Control revolves around good sanitation.

Public Health Significance: Cowpox is transmissible to people
and causes a mild infection that provides immunity to smallpox.

Contagious Ecthyma

This is an infectious pox-like disease of sheep and goats. It is
common during late summer, fall and winter.

Clinical Signs: The disease is characterized by papules that
develop into vesicles and then form a thick crust. Lesions occur
on the lips, mouth, nose and around the eyes. They may also
occur in the interdigital region and coronet. The lesions are
often fragile and bleed easily.

Diagnosis: The lesions are characteristic. The diagnosis may
be confirmed by electron microscopy.

RNA VIRUSES

Rhabdoviruses

Rhabdoviruses are single-stranded, helical RNA viruses with
a distinct bullet-shaped morphology. The enveloped virus repli-
cates in the cytoplasm of host nerve cells.

Rabies

This is a disease of all warm-blooded animals. The virus is
present in all body secretions of infected animals, including
saliva, feces, milk and urine. It is transmitted by a bite wound

that introduces the virus in saliva from infected animals. Foxes, skunks, bats and other wild animals are the principal host reservoirs. Rabies is a reportable disease that must be reported to government health authorities.

Clinical Signs: The clinical signs of rabies vary in different species. The incubation period is up to 6 months.

The prodromal phase of the disease may last 1-3 days and is usually overlooked. There is usually a change in behavior. The affected animal does not eat, seeks solitude and resents restraint. Saliva during this phase is highly infective.

In the furious form of rabies, the animal is restless and aggressive, and has excessive salivation and dilated pupils. It attacks and bites with little provocation. In males there is penile erection and females often accept copulation by males. The animal has third eyelid prolapse. Terminally, the animal shows dyspnea and dies in 2-7 days. Cats usually hide and howl.

The dumb or paralytic form of rabies is most common in dogs. This form is characterized by early paralysis of the throat and masseter muscles, and a dropped jaw. The animal is unable to eat and drink ("hydrophobia") and is not vicious. Death ensues in a few days. Cattle become agitated and can attack and bellow. Lactation stops abruptly. Affected horses have colic and often cause self-inflicted wounds.

Diagnosis: Rabies is diagnosed by the history, clinical signs, observation of inclusion bodies (*eg*, Negri bodies in nerve cells), mouse inoculation, and complement-fixation and fluorescent antibody tests.

Control: Rabies is controlled by mass vaccination of all domestic cats and dogs, and elimination of stray dogs.

An animal bitten by a rabid animal must be quarantined for 3 months if vaccinated and for 6 months if not vaccinated. Any dog biting without provocation should be kept under observation for a minimum of 14 days. If clinical signs appear, the animal will die within 10 days.

Dogs entering the United States must be accompanied by a veterinarian's certificate stating the animal has been vaccinated against rabies at least 30 days before crossing.

Public Health Significance: Rabies is transmissible to people, in which it causes essentially the same signs as in animals.

Vesicular Stomatitis

This disease resembles foot and mouth disease. In cattle and swine, excessive salivation and fever are the first signs. Vesicles appear on the oral mucosa and tongue, the skin and between the toes. In horses, tongue lesions are most pronounced.

Diagnosis: It is difficult to differentiate vesicular stomatitis from foot and mouth disease. Virus isolation from vesicular fluids and saliva is useful. Animal inoculation may be helpful in differentiating the disease (Table 1).

Control: This is a mild disease. Drastic control measures are not practiced, but it is important to isolate affected animals.

Picornaviruses

These viruses are icosahedral, have no envelope and replicate in the host cell cytoplasm.

Foot and Mouth Disease

This disease is a highly contagious disease of cloven-hooved animals and is characterized by erosive lesions in the mouth and on the muzzle and feet. The mode of transmission is by inhalation and ingestion of contaminated material.

Clinical Signs: The disease is more severe in cattle and swine. After an incubation period of 2-8 days, fever, decreased milk production, excessive salivation and vesicles in the nose and

Table 1. Species affected by 4 important viral diseases.

	Cattle	Swine	Horses
Foot and mouth disease	+	–	–
Vesicular stomatitis	+	+	+
Swine vesicular disease	–	+	–
Vesicular exanthema	–	+	–/+

mouth, and between the claws and on the coronary band of the feet are observed. After vesicles appear, there is profound salivation and lameness. Pregnant animals may abort. In swine, lameness is the first sign noted and foot lesions are usually severe.

Diagnosis: Vesicle fluid and epithelial tissue from ruptured vesicles can be used for a range of diagnostic tests. Complement fixation is useful and results are available within a few hours. Cell culture lines are used to isolate the virus. Animal inoculation is diagnostic (Table 1).

Control: Canada, the United States, Australia and the United Kingdom are free from foot and mouth disease. This was achieved by slaughter of infected and exposed animals in quarantined areas.

When foot and mouth disease is suspected, control measures include quarantine of suspected animals and area until the disease is identified, appropriate sample collection and confirmation of the disease, strict sanitation, slaughter of all affected and exposed animals and appropriate disposal of carcasses, and thorough disinfection of the premises. This is a reportable disease. Vaccination is not practiced.

Public Health Significance: People are susceptible to infection by this virus.

Vesicular Disease

This disease is characterized by vesicular lesions in the mouth and on the feet of pigs.

Clinical Signs: The first clinical sign usually noted is sudden lameness in a number of pigs in a herd, with lesions in the mouth, snout and coronary band. The affected animal's back arches and the pig may become recumbent. Transient fever and anorexia develop. The horn and sole of the hoof may slough off or separate. This differentiates the disease from foot and mouth disease and vesicular stomatitis.

Diagnosis: Various diagnostic tests are available, including animal inoculation, complement fixation and ELISA (Table 1).

Control: Vaccination is not practiced.

Caliciviruses

Caliciviruses are icosahedral, have single-stranded RNA and replicate in host cell cytoplasm. They are slightly larger than picornaviruses.

Feline Calicivirus Infection

This is another viral infection of the respiratory tract of cats. This virus causes sneezing, mild nasal discharge and ulceration of the oral mucosa, which is very painful. Affected cats do not eat until the oral lesions are healed.

Treatment and Control: Treatment is supportive and includes fluids and antibiotics. Vaccines are available in multivalent vaccines.

Reoviruses

Reoviruses have double-stranded RNA and no envelopes, are icosahedral, and replicate in host cell cytoplasm.

Blue Tongue

Blue tongue is an infectious disease of ruminants, but is most prevalent in sheep. It has not been officially reported in Canada but is transmitted by insect vectors. The disease occurs only during the fly season.

Clinical Signs: Principal clinical signs include cyanosis, edema, and erosions of the oral mucosa and tongue. The tongue becomes dark red and even purple, giving rise to the name "blue tongue." Lameness is caused by inflammation of the coronary band of the hoof.

Diagnosis: Laboratory sheep transmission or mouse transmission of disease is the most reliable diagnostic test. A fluorescent antibody test is available. Virus isolation is best done in embryonated eggs.

Rotaviruses

Rotaviruses contain double-stranded RNA, have no envelope, are icosahedral, and replicate in the host cell cytoplasm.

White Scours

Rotaviruses are the primary cause of diarrhea in calves over 4 days of age. Mixed infection with *E coli* and coronavirus are common. Overcrowding and poor hygiene contribute to severity of the disease. Death may occur due to dehydration, but animals may recover within 3-5 days.

Laboratory Diagnosis: Diagnosis is by ELISA and electron microscopy of feces and demonstration of viral particles.

Treatment and Control: Treatment is essentially the same as colibacillosis (Chapter 5). Enough colostrum ingestion is most important. Vaccination of calves may be useful.

Coronaviruses

These are single-stranded RNA viruses with pleomorphic morphology. They are circular, with ray-like "sun knobs." They are enveloped and replicate in the host cell cytoplasm.

Transmissible Gastroenteritis

This is a highly infectious disease of swine and usually seen at farrowing. It is a major clinical disease in unweaned piglets.

Clinical Signs: There is sudden onset of vomiting and foul-smelling diarrhea that often contains curds of milk. In the older pigs the infection is less severe or sometimes inapparent.

Diagnosis: The disease is diagnosed by clinical signs of sudden onset of vomiting and diarrhea, and the rapidly spreading nature of the disease. Diagnosis is confirmed by identification of viruses by electron microscopy, fluorescent antibody testing, virus isolation, and demonstration of a rising antibody titer in paired serum samples from a sow with an affected litter.

Control: Sows should be vaccinated 3 weeks before farrowing. Affected pigs should be isolated. Footwear and clothing should be changed when entering or leaving barns.

Neonatal Diarrhea in Calves

Coronaviral diarrhea occurs in calves at about 1 week of age and lasts 4-5 days. Diarrhea caused by coronavirus is not as common as diarrhea caused by rotavirus.

Feline Infectious Peritonitis

Clinical Signs: Affected cats are anorexic and depressed, and have a fever. In the classical wet form for the disease, there is abdominal distension by accumulation of peritoneal fluid with a high protein content. Affected cats usually die within 1-8 weeks.

Diagnosis: A fluorescent antibody test is available. Virus isolation is used to confirm the diagnosis.

Treatment and Control: Treatment is supportive and consists of fluids, antibiotics, corticosteroids and peritoneal lavage. Infected cats must be isolated. Cats showing antibodies to the virus must be regarded as infected.

Paramyxoviruses

These are pleomorphic single-stranded RNA viruses that replicate in host cell cytoplasm. The viral envelope has short projections.

Canine Distemper

This is a deadly infectious diseases of dogs. It can affect dogs of any age but is most common in puppies, especially stressed puppies. Transmission is usually by inhalation.

Clinical Signs: Clinical signs begin as gastrointestinal disturbance. The animal is anorexic, and vomiting and diarrhea soon develop. There are fever and conjunctivitis. The disease may also have a respiratory and/or a nervous component.

Diagnosis: Clinical signs are not diagnostic. Laboratory diagnosis is necessary. Immunofluorescence of antigen on impression smears of conjunctival samples or lymphocytes is useful.

Treatment and Control: Treatment consists of supportive therapy and antibiotics to control secondary infections. Affected dogs should be isolated. Many types of vaccines are available.

Canine Parainfluenza

This virus contributes to kennel cough (see Tracheobronchitis). Modified-live-virus vaccines included in multivalent vaccines are available for prevention.

Equine Influenza

This is a very contagious respiratory disease especially prevalent in racehorses and show horses. It is commonly known as "flu" or "cough" and is not a serious disease but is notable because it affects the animal's performance. The disease is spread by inhalation.

Clinical Signs: Affected horses have a fever up to 41 C, a dry hacking cough, and slight, watery nasal discharge. Horses may recover in 1-2 weeks if they are unstressed. Secondary bacterial infection can result in pneumonia.

Control: In an outbreak, the premises should be kept under quarantine for at least 4 weeks. After all horses have recovered, the premises should be cleaned and disinfected. Horses should be vaccinated within 6-12 weeks before a show or race season. High-risk horses should be vaccinated every 3-4 months.

Togaviruses

Togaviruses are single-stranded RNA viruses. They are icosahedral, have envelopes and replicate in host cell cytoplasm.

Equine Encephalomyelitis

This is a viral encephalitis of horses of North America. Three strains of the virus are involved: Eastern, Western and Venezuelan. The disease is transmitted by insect bites, especially by the *Culex* species of mosquito. The disease incidence is highest where the mosquito population is greatest.

Clinical Signs: After an incubation period of 1-3 days, fever, anorexia and depression may progress to nervous signs. Horses may walk into objects, walk in circles, or show incoordination. The head is hung low, and the horse appears asleep. This may be followed by paralysis and death.

Laboratory Diagnosis: Diagnosis is by isolation of virus from blood and brain tissue, and inoculation of guinea pigs.

Treatment and Control: Supportive therapy and good nursing care are helpful in mild cases of disease. Mosquito control also helps minimize disease. A vaccine is available and is often combined with tetanus vaccine.

Public Health Significance: Eastern encephalomyelitis is more severe in people than the Western type. It causes signs ranging from a mild flu-like syndrome to encephalitis.

Bovine Viral Diarrhea

This disease is most common in cattle 8 months to 2 years old. The disease also can occur in calves and is transmitted by direct contact.

Clinical Signs: Clinical signs include depression, anorexia, bloat, fever, increased heart and respiratory rates, and profuse foul-smelling diarrhea. The feces may contain mucus and blood. Oral lesions occur in 5-10% of affected cattle. In pregnant cows, the virus may cause fetal death, mummification, abortion, or congenital cerebral, ocular or musculoskeletal defects.

Diagnosis: Clinical signs, history and postmortem findings are diagnostic in severe cases. Virus isolation is also useful.

Treatment and Control: Treatment consists of supportive fluid therapy and good nursing care. An effective vaccine is available.

Newcastle Disease

Newcastle disease is a series of clinical entities in domestic poultry and other birds, ranging from inapparent infection to a fulminating fatal disease. The form is determined by the strain of virus involved.

The mild form of Newcastle disease is characterized by transitory respiratory illness and interruption of egg production. Moderately affected birds show incoordination and other nervous signs. The severe form of Newcastle disease has high mortality. It is characterized by severe respiratory signs, with coughing, sneezing, cessation of egg production and watery green diarrhea. Nervous signs include walking in circles, walking backward, and twisting of the head and neck. In North America, the mild form is most common.

Diagnosis: Diagnosis is by virus isolation from samples of spleen, brain and lungs, or by allantoic inoculation. The hemagglutination inhibition test can detect antibody.

Control: A modified-live vaccine is administered by dust, spray or via drinking water.

Public Health Significance: The Newcastle virus causes conjunctivitis in people.

Rinderpest

This is a highly infectious disease, characterized by necrosis and erosion of the mucosa in digestive and respiratory tracts of ruminants.

Clinical Signs: After an incubation period of 4-15 days, affected animals show high fever, anorexia, depression, increased salivation and a nasal discharge. Necrotic pinpoint to cheesy plaque-like lesions are found on the gums, oral mucosa and tongue. In the final stages, diarrhea may be watery and contain mucus and blood. Death occurs within 6-12 days. This disease is not seen in North America.

Diagnosis: Diagnosis is by virus isolation.

Control: In countries free of rinderpest, measures are designed to prevent introduction of the disease. In enzootic areas, a vaccination program is useful.

References
Chapters 27-30

1. Blood DC *et al*: *Veterinary Medicine*. 6th ed. Bailliere Tindall, London, 1983.

2. Fenner F *et al*: *Veterinary Virology*. Academic Press, Orlando, FL, 1987.

3. Fraser CM *et al*: *The Merck Veterinary Manual*. 8th ed. Merck, Rahway, NJ, 1986.

4. Tindall JF *et al*: *Hagan and Bruner's Microbiology and Infectious Diseases of Domestic Animals*. 8th ed. Cornell Univ Press, Ithaca, NY, 1988.

5. Roberts WA and Carter GR: *Essentials of Veterinary Virology*. Michigan State Univ Press, East Lansing, MI, 1981.

Glossary

Active Immunity: Immunity produced by the body during specific infection or by inoculation of vaccines.

Acute Disease: Rapid development of clinical illness, reaching the peak and ending fairly quickly.

Aerial Mycelium: The part of fungal hyphae that projects above the culture medium.

Agglutination: Visible clumping or aggregation of cells or particles as a result of the reaction between antigen and specific antibody.

Alpha Hemolysis: Partial lysis of red blood cells resulting in a greenish or slimy appearance around bacterial colonies on blood agar.

Antibiotic: Organic compound produced by a microorganism that inhibits growth of another organism.

Antibody (Immunoglobulin): Serum proteins produced by an animal in response to introduction of an antigen.

Antigen: An agent, when introduced into an animal's body, that stimulates production of antibodies.

Antitoxin: Antibody to a toxin that can react with and neutralize the specific toxin.

Ascus: Sac-like structure containing ascospores developed during sexual reproduction.

Attenuation: Procedure by which the pathogenicity of a given organism is reduced.

Bacteremia: Presence of bacteria in the blood.

Bacteriophage: Virus that infects bacterial cells.

Beta Hemolysis: Complete hemolysis around bacterial colonies on blood agar.

Carrier: Animal that, without showing signs of the disease, harbors the specific pathogens and may disseminate them.

Chronic Disease: Condition of slow onset in which signs exist for a prolonged period.

Coagulase: Enzyme produced by pathogenic staphylococci that causes coagulation of plasma.

Colony: Macroscopically visible growth of microorganisms on solid culture medium. Each colony is a pure culture.

Conidiophore: Specialized fungal hypha on which conidia develop singly or in groups.

Conidium (Aleuriospore, Conidiospore): An asexual fungal spore produced on a specialized structure known as a conidiophore.

Contagious Disease: Infectious disease transferable from one host to another.

Culture: Growth of a particular organism on or in medium under controlled conditions.

Dimorphism: Ability of fungi to grow as filamentous forms or reproduce, depending on conditions of growth.

Eclipse Period: Time between initial virus infection and the appearance of new infective virus particles.

Ectothrix: Formation of fungal spores outside an infected hair shaft.

Endogenous Infection: Infection produced within or caused by microorganisms within an animal's body.

Endothrix: Formation of fungal spores within an infected hair shaft.

Epizootic: Occurrence of a disease affecting large numbers of animals within a short time, and usually spreading rapidly.

Etiologic Agent: Agent causing disease.

Exogenous Infection: Infection originating outside or caused by outside factors.

Fusiform: Spindle shaped.

Gamma Hemolysis: No hemolysis caused by bacterial colonies on blood agar.

Gelatin: Protein derived from skin, hair, bones and tendons that is used in culture media.

Germ Tube: Tube-like process growing out of a germinating fungal spore that eventually develops into the mycelium.

Hyphae: Filaments that compose the mycelium of a fungus.

Immunity: Relative protection of an animal against infection.

Immunodeficiency: A state of impaired immune function.

Imperfect Fungi: Fungi that apparently lack the sexual means of reproduction, and that reproduce asexually.

Incubation Period: Period after a pathogen enters the body and before signs of illness appear.

Infection: Process whereby pathogenic organisms enter and multiply in the tissues of an animsl's body.

Infectious (Communicable) Disease: Disease transferable from one host to another.

Labile: Unstable or readily changed by physical, chemical or biologic processes.

Lysis: Rupture of a cell.

Macroconidium: Large, usually multicellular fungal conidium.

Macroscopic: Capable of observation with the naked eye.

Mastitis: Inflammation of udder or mammary glands.

Microconidium: Small, single-celled fungal conidium.

Monomorphic: Fungi that grow and reproduce in only the mold form or yeast form.

Morbidity: Proportion of animals becoming clinically ill after infection.

Mortality: Proportion of deaths in a group of sick animals.

Mycelium: Tangled mass of fungal hyphae.

Mycosis: Disease caused by a fungus.

Natural Immunity: Immunity that is inherited genetically.

Necrosis: Death of cells or tissue in a localized area.

Negri Bodies: Acidophilic, intracytoplasmic inclusion bodies that develop in nerve cells of animals with rabies.

Noncontagious Disease: Disease usually transmitted by a vector.

Nuclease: Enzyme capable of splitting nucleic acid.

Panzootic: Widespread outbreak of disease.

Passive Immunity: Short-term immunity produced by transfer of preformed antibodies.

Pellicle: Film of microorganisms on the surface of a broth culture.

Perfect Fungi: Fungi that have sexual and asexual means of reproduction.

Prodromal Stage: Onset of signs of illness at the end of the incubation period.

Pure Culture: Population of microorganisms consisting of only a single species.

Purulent: Consisting of pus.

Pus: A fluid produced as a result of inflammation, mainly composed of leukocytes, serum and debris.

Quarantine: Limitation of movement of an animal exposed to a communicable disease to prevent contact with those not exposed.

Racquet Hyphae: Vegetative fungal hyphae with terminal swelling of segments, resembling a tennis racquet.

Rhizoid: Radiating, root-like fungal hyphae arising at the nodes of *Rhizopus*.

Saprophyte: Organism living on dead or decaying organic matter.

Septate Hyphae: Fungal hyphae with cross walls or septa.

Spherules: Spherical multinucleated cells of *Coccidioides*.

Spores: Reproductive structures formed asexually or sexually by microoganisms.

Thallus: Fungal colony readily recognized by its fuzzy cottony appearance made up of mycelium.

Titer: Level of antibodies in the blood to a specific microbial pathogen.

Toxemia: Condition in which toxins are liberated by bacteria and circulated in the blood.

Toxoid: Toxin modified to eliminate its toxicity but not its ability to stimulate antibody production.

Tuberculin: Growth products of, or specific substances extracted from, *Mycobacterium tuberculosis*, used to diagnose tuberculosis.

Vegetative Mycelium: The part of fungal hyphae that projects above the culture medium.

Viropexis: Attachment of a virus to an animal cell membrane, and subsequent engulfment by the cell.

Virulence: Degree of pathogenicity.

Index

A

Absidia, 165
Actinobacillus species, 95-97
Actinomyces, 115, 116
adenoviruses, 187, 188
aerobes, 99-104
anaerobes, 57-59, 85-97
antimicrobial susceptibility
 tests, 54-56
Arizona, 90
aseptic technique, 36
Aspergillus, 165, 166

B

bacilli, 73-79, 81-84, 85-97, 99-104
Bacillus species, 73-75
bacteria, *Actinobacillus,* 95-97
 Actinomyces, 115, 116
 aerobes, 99-104
 anaerobes, 57-59, 85-97
 antimicrobial susceptibility, 54-56
 Arizona, 90
 arrangement, 14
 bacilli, 73-79, 81-97, 99-104
 Bacillus, 73-75
 Bacteroides, 108, 109
 Bordetella, 102
 Borrelia, 129, 130
 Brucella, 100-102
 Campylobacter, 111-114
 capsule, 15, 16
 cell membrane, 17

cell wall, 16, 17
Chlamydia, 132
classification, 11, 12
Clostridium, 75-80
cocci, 63-72, 105, 106
coccobacilli, 105, 106
colony characteristics, 39, 40
Corynebacterium, 120-123
Coxiella, 131, 132
culture, 32-40
cytoplasm, 17
Dermatophilus, 116, 117
diseases, 5-9
endospores, 20, 21
enzymes, 6
Erysipelothrix, 82-84
Escherichia coli, 85-87
Eubacterium, 123
fimbriae, 19
flagella, 18, 19
Francisella, 103, 104
Fusobacterium, 107, 108
Gram-negative, 48-54, 85-97,
 99-104, 105, 106, 107-109
Gram-positive, 46-48, 63-72,
 73-79, 81-84
growth, 22-27
Hemophilus, 93-95
identification, 43-54
infection, 5-9
intracellular, 131, 132
Klebsiella, 90
laboratory procedures, 29-61
Lancefield groups, 66, 67